The Teacher's Guide to
ACCESSIBLE YOGA

BEST PRACTICES FOR SHARING YOGA WITH EVERY BODY

The Teacher's Guide to

ACCESSIBLE

**BEST PRACTICES
FOR SHARING YOGA
WITH EVERY BODY** YOGA

Jivana Heyman

Foreword by Anjali Rao
Photos by Sarit Z. Rogers

RAINBOW MIND PUBLICATIONS

First Edition
Printed in the United States of America

Cover design by Deanna Michalopoulos
Interior design by **Booknook.biz**

ISBN
979-8-9896800-0-9 (paperback)
979-8-9896800-1-6 (ebook)

To my students, who are my teachers

CONTENTS

Part Three: Teaching Subtle Practices

ACKNOWLEDGMENTS

IT FEELS LIKE a divine coincidence that I'm finishing writing this book on the anniversary of the death of my best friend, Kurt, who died of AIDS in 1995. After all, he was the one who encouraged me to become a yoga teacher. In fact, I finished my yoga teacher training just months before he passed, and here he is again, supporting and guiding me.

What I most want to share is my endless gratitude and appreciation for the yoga teachings, which are an indigenous practice of the people of South Asia. They have been kept alive as a living history for thousands of years with tremendous love and care. It's essential to honor both the well-known teachers as well as the unknown practitioners and teachers who have kept these teachings alive for so long.

I also appreciate you for stepping into this ancient stream of yoga with me. If you're here wading in the shallows or diving deep, I know that you share my heartfelt gratitude for the wisdom and expansiveness of these teachings.

Thank you to my husband, Matt, who has been by my side for thirty years, as well as our kids, Charlie and Violet, and our family: Charles Mary, Judy Raboy, and my siblings and their partners: Jenny, Mike, Tim, Olya, Chris, Anna, Amanda and Greg, and all their kids, Izzy, Ollie, Eli, Aaron, Caleb, Cooper, Dylan, Dash, Noah, and Rose.

So much gratitude to my ancestors, in particular my mother and father, and my grandmother, Shirley Kent, who was my first yoga teacher. Gratitude to all of my incredible teachers, especially Kazuko Onodera, who took me under her wing and showed me the power of yoga when I most needed it.

Thank you to everyone who was involved with this project, especially Brina Lord for managing it all, Deanna Michalopoulos for the cover design, endless support, and memes. Special thanks to my incredible editor, Kat Rebar. Also, thanks to the Accessible Yoga team which includes Zane Ali, Robyn Bell, Tan Hubbard-Hood, and Raeeka Yassaie. Special thanks to M Camellia for contributing to the section on agency and consent, and all their support.

Thank you to Sarit Z. Rogers for her photography and friendship, as well as our incredible models, Gustavo Ritterstein, Aurora M. Ruiz, and Robin Schievink. The class that we did together felt like the perfect example of an Accessible Yoga class, and that comes through in the photos.

Thank you to Seth Powell, PhD, for letting me reference his research and use his photo of the Yoga Narasimha with a strap. Special thanks to all the contributors, including Indu Arora, Judith Lasater, Shanna Small, Michelle Cassandra Johnson, M Camellia, Tristan Katz, Jason Crandell, Avery Kalapa, Nityda Gessel, Shawn Moore, Melissa Shah, Tracee Stanley, and Kino MacGregor.

Gratitude to Anjali Rao for writing the beautiful foreword, and for the gift of her friendship and wisdom. I'm endlessly grateful to Anjali for leading the Accessible Yoga Association Board, and to all of our board members: Ashley Williams, Colin Lieu, Sunny Barbee, Priya Wagner, Tristan Katz, Reggie Hubbard, Ryan McGraw, Sarani Fedman, Tamika Caston-Miller, Avery Kalapa, and Rodrigo Souza.

Grateful for the love and support from Amber Karnes (and for her contribution to the section on yoga for larger bodies), kelley nicole palmer, Swami Ramananda, ML Maitreyi, Cheri Clampett, Matthew Pesendian, Rachelle Knowles, Beth Frankl, Kalyani Baral, Linda

Sparrowe, Adrian Molina, Marc Morozumi, Susanna Barkataki, De Jur Jones, Chinnamasta Stiles, Matthew Sanford, and David Lipsius. Thank you to Joel, Sayde, and the team at Launch My Book. Also, thank you to the 2023 cohort of our Accessible Yoga Teacher Training program for inspiring much of what I share here.

I feel so incredibly grateful for the Accessible Yoga Community and for all of our Ambassadors around the world, sharing the message of equity in yoga.

[Note: In some of the translations of ancient texts that I quote, I have replaced the gendered language that is used to represent the divine with neutral pronouns. My goal is to make these texts more accessible and modernize the translations.]

FOREWORD

"ONE LAMP can never light another unless it continues to burn its own flame," said Rabindranath Tagore, the Nobel Peace laureate and beloved humanist who is revered by millions for his revolutionary perspective about education, which emphasized experiential learning and agency of the student. A teacher is first and foremost a student of what they are teaching—someone who consistently, with *shraddha* (dedication) is honing their skill in all ways possible. As teachers, we excavate from our lived experiences, transmute our mistakes into lessons, listen to our hearts, and share all of this as a gift to our students.

To teach is to serve. This is what I have been taught by my own teachers, and it's what anchors my approach to teaching as *seva* (service). To teach yoga is to change the world—one student, maybe even one class, at a time. Even though yoga consists of a diverse and often paradoxical system of teachings, one can agree that yoga is a practice of both individual and collective transformation.

The practice and the teachings of yoga invite us into an unveiling of who we are—our human, whole, and messy selves. We connect with our body, unveil our embedded *samskaras* and our cultural conditioning so we know ourselves better. As teachers, we shine a light to help our students navigate their own paths. Yoga is ultimately a process of self-discovery. As conduits of this ancient wisdom, we have a tremendous responsibility to shoulder. We influence others' lives in profound ways, and thus need to be as prepared as we can for this pivotal role.

The ancient *gurukul* system, where students lived with a teacher for nearly a decade so the students could imbibe everything from yoga to archery to logic, has shifted now. Back then, the teacher would intuit and glean from each student what they need to learn, and share that either based on the student's future role in the community, innate disposition, *prakruti* (ayurvedic constitution), or talent. The student-teacher relationship was thus deemed an intensely personal and sacred one—one where immense reverence was bestowed upon the guru.

There are many stories about the exalted status accorded to teachers in the Vedas, Upanishads, Puranas, and the great epics the Mahabharata and the Ramayana. Traditionally, this relationship has been hierarchical and rather formal. The teacher could and did test the readiness of the student to receive the teachings. Many were turned away if they failed to meet the standards set forth by the guru. And yes, some of these stories portray the teachers as complicated and flawed beings.

For example, Dronacharya, the mighty teacher of the Pandavas and the Kauravas in the Bhagavad Gita, refused to teach a young, talented archer, named Ekalavya because he was from a tribal community and not from the princely or the scholarly class. The story ends in heartbreak as he demands the sacrifice of Ekalavya's right thumb to ensure he never surpasses Arjuna as the most proficient archer in the land. This story teaches us many things: how we can disrupt hierarchy and classism as teachers, and how we have to practice discernment as students.

The socioeconomic context of yoga has changed drastically today, where group classes are the norm and the teacher-student relationship is not as prolonged or in-depth as it used to be. As teachers of modern yoga, we have to conscientiously learn how to keep our students safe and supported in all the ways that they need.

This book is a much needed tool for those who aspire to teach yoga in all its expansiveness—as a way of life rather than just as a physical practice. Jivana invites the reader into all the myriad and often intimidating aspects of teaching with a gentle-yet-fierce discernment of our positions as teachers in the yoga community—as people who can contour the containers for another's experience of their body and mind, while simultaneously steering our own paths as imperfect, embodied beings.

Jivana writes not only from his immense teaching experience but also from his role as an influential thought leader who is shifting the narrative of ableism and individualism in modern Western yoga. His insight into yoga stems from an unwavering curiosity, continued learning, and love for the practice that he often says saved his life at a very critical time.

He is steadfast in his commitment to uplift other teachers, something that I find unique and endearing in the hypercompetitive world that we live in today. As someone who has had the pleasure and the honor of working with Jivana closely, I have seen this collaborative and open approach first hand—an approach that is reflected in the book as well.

My sincere wish is that this book inspires, educates, and motivates all those who are on the threshold of sharing the teachings of yoga in any way and that it continues to illuminate your ongoing journey as a teacher and a practitioner. This is how we serve the world we live in, one student at a time.

—Anjali Rao

INTRODUCTION

BEFORE COVID, I had the incredible good fortune to travel all over the world training yoga teachers. It was a dream job that I had worked toward for decades. One challenge that quickly became apparent was the language barrier that I faced in many countries. I'm only comfortable teaching in English, even though I can speak a little French and Spanish. So, I found communication to be an issue at many of my programs. Translators were amazingly helpful, but there was a limit to what they could do.

In 2013, I was invited to teach my Accessible Yoga Training at an ashram in Austria, which attracted students from all over Europe. That meant that the forty-plus students in my training all spoke different languages. I was thrilled to be traveling to this amazing country to spend time practicing and teaching at an ashram nestled in the alps. I was impressed by the massive gray mountain peaks all around, but it was the bright blue sky, white clouds, and green grass that really mesmerized me.

It seemed like everything was brighter at that altitude, or maybe it was the brightness that comes from all the deep practice that had been shared in that sacred space. I was excited, but also very nervous to be teaching there. It dawned on me that I had never taught such a diverse language group, and I couldn't figure out how we would communicate with each other. I did have a German translator, but for the other languages I was on my own.

During the training, I ask the students to break up into small groups to practice teaching to each other. It occurred to me that I could divide the groups up by language so they could teach each other in the language of their choosing. So we ended up with small groups teaching in German, French, Spanish, Italian, and English. We only had one large lecture hall to use, so this was all happening at the same time in the same space. It was very chaotic, and I was worried that it wouldn't work.

I vividly remember walking around the room and listening to yoga being taught in five different languages simultaneously. At first I tried to get the translator to help me decipher what each person was saying, but it wasn't possible because so many people were teaching at the same time.

Finally, I sat down in the middle of the room exasperated. I needed to find another way. As I sat there listening to words I didn't understand, I tried to let go and allow the sounds to wash over me. As I relaxed into the moment, I realized that I could feel the yoga being shared. Each group was engaged in their practice, and it was easy to see that yoga was happening beyond the words. Not only could I see it, I could feel it. All the teachers were opening to the power of the teachings and sharing their hearts with each other.

That experience reminded me of how powerful the teachings are, and that teaching is so much bigger than us as individuals. It also completely changed the way I observe yoga teachers when I'm training them. I realized that I could sense the yoga beyond the details of the words someone chose.

Yoga is more of an art than a science and, like all art, I could connect to the energy of the experience by listening with my heart instead of my head. Working in this way, I found that I could give very specific feedback to teachers, even if I didn't speak their language and I had no idea what they were actually saying. For example,

I could feel when someone was withdrawn, or overly enthusiastic. I could sense the responsiveness of the students, and feel whether they were connected or disengaged.

This is not to say that words aren't incredibly important since language is the medium of teaching, but there is a lot more to teaching than what comes out of our mouths. In the end, I saw that so much of yoga teaching happens on an energetic level which makes sense since yoga is an energetic practice. This gave me insight into ways to truly make yoga accessible—beyond words.

Sometimes it can be difficult to describe the subtle shifts in energy necessary to make yoga equitable and accessible, but that's my goal in this book. Teaching yoga is a complex and subtle combination of skills. We need to be knowledgeable about teaching methodology, anatomy and physiology, yoga philosophy and history, business management, accounting, marketing, contract law, and so much more. It can often feel like too much for just one person! In the end, the most important quality in a teacher is their love and dedication to the practice.

Support Along the Path

While the essence of yoga hasn't changed over millennia, the way yoga is taught has continued to change. Yoga evolved in ashrams, with wandering sadhus, and in the daily life of South Asian communities. There was a cultural context for the practice. Then as yoga moved to the West, it was packaged and appropriated. We were told to focus on physical achievement when, in fact, this was in direct opposition to the spiritual goals of the practice.

Often the heart of yoga was hidden by capitalist influences which focused on competition and profit. Even so, the heart of yoga was unchanged. It may have been hidden, but it was never erased. Our challenge today is figuring out how to share the traditional essence of the practice in a way that is respectful to its ancient lineage and still pertinent to contemporary practitioners.

While the essence of yoga hasn't changed—it's still about spiritual awakening—what has changed is the form the practice takes and the way it is taught. Methods that were common even twenty years ago are no longer considered acceptable. Just a few years ago, it was not uncommon for yoga teachers to yell, criticize, make fun of, or degrade their students in public classes.

Even worse, there are way too many examples of teachers who physically or sexually abused their students. In fact, it was often the most famous teachers who were the most abusive, such as Bikram Choudhry (Bikram Yoga), Pattabhi Jois (Ashtanga Yoga), or Yogi Bhajan (3HO Kundalini Yoga). My teacher, Swami Satchidananda, is included on this list, so I am very familiar with the dangers found in many traditional lineages. This abuse is not only upsetting; it also challenges us to find ways to teach that don't allow this aspect of our tradition to continue.

Practicing What We Preach

Tirumalai Krishnamacharya is often referred to as the father of modern yoga, although I think modern yoga actually has many parents. There is a famous quote attributed to him that says, "If you can breathe, you can do yoga." With that one sentence he challenged all of us to rethink the way we are teaching and the contents of our classes.

Today we are standing at a crossroads in the history of yoga. This is a moment that asks us to practice what we preach and to embody the teachings of yoga in the way we teach. It seems like such a simple, and even obvious question, but how many yoga teachers are truly living according to the teachings that they share? I know that it's a constant struggle and daily commitment for me.

In order for us to move forward in a way that is both respectful to the tradition of yoga and cognizant of our students' innate humanity and agency, we need to bring a fresh eye to the way we're teaching. It's clear that yoga teaching methodology has changed over millennia, and much of that is in response to the cultural norms where yoga has been taught. While we still have a long way to go, my hope is that teachers today are ready to unite yoga's ancient spiritual calling and a love of humanity.

Working together, we can create a yoga community that doesn't allow for abuse of any kind to continue, and we can build a community of yoga teachers who respect their students' boundaries and strive to lift their students up, rather than to push them down.

The problem is, as yoga teachers, we often don't have the resources and support we need to continue evolving. We need to find ways to continue to study and practice so that our skills evolve and our classes can be truly safe and appropriate for this moment. To be honest, the lack of evolution in our teaching practice is not really our fault. It's the result of a very limited yoga teacher training system that is failing to keep up with the times.

Most yoga teachers I know are incredible people who are truly dedicated to the practice and want to serve with their whole heart (and I love you for that!). This book is a message of hope that comes out of my gratitude for all of your service. It's also a quick education in what you need to know right now. With this additional knowledge and skill, you can make your classes welcoming and safe for anyone who is interested in practicing yoga.

The Road Ahead

The work involved in making yoga accessible includes reflecting on your role in the classroom, issues of power and consent, cultural appropriation, trauma-sensitive teaching, physical accessibility, and much more. To effectively communicate with your students, you need to educate yourself around the cultural issues that they are facing, and consider how those issues show up in your classes. For example, learning how to address racism, ableism, and transphobia in your classes can allow the heart of yoga to shine through in your teaching. Otherwise, these issues become barriers to safety and to learning.

As practitioners, yoga asks us to continually reflect on our own minds—on our words and actions. Our practice demands that we step back and think about the way we are teaching, the way we share power with our students, as well as our relationship to the teachings. It's easy to take a yoga teacher training, do what you are told to do by your teachers, and then repeat the same phrases and cues over and over without really thinking about what you're saying or teaching. It's also easy to take a yoga teacher training and then have no idea how to share the teachings with real people with real bodies and real problems.

I've seen so many lives transformed by yoga, including my own, and I've dedicated my life to making these teachings accessible to anyone who's interested in them. My last two books both focus on the same themes that I address here, but in a slightly different way. In those books, I've only referred to teaching in passing, rather than focusing on the details of the thing I love most in the world—teaching yoga!

I see that yoga teachers are truly on the front lines of a major transformation in the world. We hold in our hands the tools to change lives, and in turn, entire communities. The potential is really awe-inspiring. But sometimes, I worry about how we're wielding that power. The question is: Are you teaching in a way that lifts people up and shows them their own beauty and potential, or are you teaching in a way that makes people feel diminished, disempowered, or unworthy?

A Yoga Teacher's Companion

This book is not exactly a yoga teacher training manual. Rather, it's a companion on the journey of becoming a yoga teacher, or continuing along the path of teaching for those of you who have been doing it for a long time. We all need support, encouragement, and inspiration at some point on this path. I know that I do, which is why I'm including the voices of so many other yoga teachers here.

In each chapter, I've asked someone who I admire to share their personal reflection on that topic. These contributions speak to the need for us all to have multiple teachers, and to be learning from multiple sources, as I am trying to do. I encourage you to read the contributor's words and consider looking them up and studying with them if you found their teaching useful.

I interviewed each of the contributors to this book by starting with one specific question related to the topics of each chapter. I have included direct quotes from them at the beginning of each chapter, and I'm also going to be releasing a podcast of these original interviews to accompany this book.

I truly hope you will take the time to listen to this series of short podcast interviews with this incredible collection of yoga teachers to hear more about their perspectives. Often the conversations quickly went much further and deeper than I could include in this book. Yoga is truly an endless topic with so much space for exploration and contemplation. That is why I've shared reflection questions throughout the book and further reflections at the end of each chapter. I hope this book is more of a conversation than a lecture, and that these prompts encourage you to respond to what I've offered here.

I'm always excited when I meet other yoga teachers, and I could literally talk with them about teaching for hours on end. This is why my husband refuses to join me if I'm meeting up with another yoga teacher! He always says, "You're going to be talking about yoga aren't you?"

I find a balance of solace and learning in all my interactions with other teachers, and I hope to share some of that in this book. This is a path that has brought me more joy and growth than I could have imagined possible. My hope is that this book will be a companion for you on your yoga teaching path as you continue to grow.

I also hope that you will expand the pool of people who you consider to be your teachers. I appreciate the wisdom that I was taught, which was to dig one deep well instead of many shallow ones. So I spent the majority of my time studying and practicing in one lineage. But, as I matured as a teacher, I was inspired by other teachers and other traditions, and they often challenged the things I had learned, and how I was teaching them. Listening to other perspectives on these teachings has greatly expanded my understanding and awe of them. That is why I find it so important to constantly seek out new teachers and new voices.

There is so much diversity within the yoga teaching world. There is power vinyasa, slow flow, hot, hatha, yin, restorative, and so many more. Each style demands different things from the teacher and, in turn, need to be adapted in different ways to become accessible. In this book, I'm trying to offer general guidance, but not everything is applicable to every style. I hope you can take what is useful for you and leave the rest.

I do not pretend to have all the answers, and I don't think you need to either. In fact, a huge part of making yoga accessible is the recognition of our own personal limitations and the cultivation of a community that will both support us when we're confused or down and also keep things real. In many ways, yoga is a practice of community. It is such a paradox because we think of yoga as an extremely personal, inner practice, yet it is by turning within that we can connect with others and truly experience our shared humanity and spirituality.

Yoga teaching has allowed me to survive, and often thrive, in a life that has held many obstacles and challenges. My prayer is that you will also benefit from the blessings of yoga, and then return the gift by sharing these beautiful practices and teachings with all of your students.

PART ONE

PREPARING TO TEACH

CHAPTER ONE

TEACH WHAT YOU LOVE

It's important for yoga practitioners, teachers, therapists, and educators to keep in mind that yoga is a philosophy first. When we think of it only as techniques, we're making it something mechanical.

Ask yourself these questions about yoga: Is it making me reflect? Is it making me curious? Is it making me inquire? Is it building self inquiry? Is it building critical thinking, which is really heavily emphasized upon in yoga, as discernment, as viveka khyati? Is it adding this everyday pause, reflection, contemplation, self inquiry, discernment? Inquiries like these are so important, because even if you're able to reach your hands to your toes, it doesn't mean that you've reached anywhere in yoga.

I'm a student on this path, and I know for sure in this lifetime my role is that of a student. From the outside it might not always look that way; I will temporarily have other roles in life, but internally, in my mind and in my heart, my role as student is absolutely clear. Just study, just dedicate your lifetime to studying this. If I don't do it honestly and sincerely, then the loss is mine because yoga has so much to offer. Most of us are just walking out of yoga class with flexibility and strength. And as teachers, maybe we are also walking out with some money.

But yoga has a promise that is bigger than life. It has a promise that's called absolute freedom.

I think it's important to know that when we fail to see and embrace this, it's not yoga's loss. It's our loss. Yoga is not a person who is going to be mad at you. Yoga is not a person who is going to hold something against you. Yoga is a timeless body of wisdom. And we are the ones who lose out if we are not understanding the depth, the capacity, the breadth of it. We're making a bad deal with yoga.

Irrespective of the language that you use or how it may look on the outside, all yoga is subtle. Yoga is philosophy first, technique later. Regardless of the technique you're using, it's an external shell. It's important to ask: Are your words and your silence communicating the heart of yoga? Are you giving people resources to come back to themselves? Reminding people of the realization that we may be going through grief, something may be broken in our life, but we are still whole. There is nothing that is needed from outside to make us whole.

—Indu Arora

IN THE 1990s, I started teaching yoga so that I could share these practices with my community of people with HIV and AIDS. We were in the middle of the AIDS epidemic, and many of my students were sick and dying. What my students and I learned together was that yoga gave us accessible and powerful tools for healing on a deep mental, emotional, and spiritual level.

A few of my students taught me a lesson that was truly life-changing: Yoga could provide them healing even when they were dying. I remember one student, who was near death, telling me something that really stuck with me. He explained, "I'm grateful that I got so sick because it led me on a spiritual journey back to myself." Amazingly, that student ended up getting better. I just wish we could learn these lessons without so much suffering.

Since then, I've been trying to honor their legacy by sharing this message of hope with the yoga community, and with the general public. The message is that yoga is not about physical achievement or even physical healing; yoga is about a deep internal spiritual connection, and it's available to all of us at any time in our journey.

What's really remarkable about yoga is that it allows us to engage every aspect of our being—our body, our breath, our mind, and our actions—in our spiritual journey. This is unusual since most contemporary spiritual practices don't include such powerful techniques for incorporating the body. Yoga is an embodied spiritual practice that allows the body to flow in the moving prayer of asana. But we can't let the beauty and power of asana fool us. Yoga is not really about the body at all.

The truth of yoga is that the body and mind are temporary, constantly changing, and mortal. Our main job as yoga practitioners is to connect to our spirit which is immortal, everlasting, and pure. This is the lesson of the Bhagavad Gita, where Sri Krishna explains:

> You were never born; you will never die. You have never changed; you can never change. Unborn, eternal, immutable, immemorial, you do not die when the body dies.[1]

I'm bringing this up in the beginning of this book so that you can reflect on the way you are currently practicing and teaching yoga before you consider how to make it accessible. Unfortunately, when we overly simplify yoga to be just about the poses, we strip it of its most essential meaning. We appropriate the practice from its traditional roots in South Asia and turn it into a commodity to be sold by capitalist interests.

So the issue is more than just one of respect and care for continuing the ancient legacy of the yoga lineage. It's about holding these precious teachings in a way that respects their purpose, their background, and their proper application.

In order to do so, we need to consider the fullness of the practice. The essential teaching of yoga is that we all share the same spiritual essence no matter what our background or ability may be. We share the same essence whether we have a disability, or a larger body, or if we're an older adult, or if we're a child. In fact, as we discover how deeply we are all connected, we not only grow to accept each other's differences but to genuinely celebrate them. That is the basis of equity in yoga—a celebration of the diversity of our bodies, minds, and experiences, as we simultaneously explore our deep, undeniable, and unbreakable connection.

In order to make this concept a reality, we have got to let go of the idea of complex asana equating advanced yoga. There really is no correlation between our physical ability and the depth of our spiritual connection. This is why I always say that if it's not accessible, it's not yoga—because we all have equal access to the heart of yoga, and we all deserve a practice that allows us to unite with our spirit within.

Tradition & Innovation

Most people think that adapting yoga is a very contemporary thing to do, and sometimes I hear concerns that something is lost when we adapt the practice. But it is possible to find examples of adaptive practice in some of the most ancient images of asana that exist. The *yogapaṭṭa*, or yoga strap, can be found in ancient sculptures of yoga asana from over 2000 years ago. According to research by yoga historian Seth Powell:

> *Many aspects of modern postural yoga are clearly just that: modern innovations. The concept of a large group yoga class, the majority demographic of female teachers and practitioners, and*

indeed, much of the vinyāsa "flow" style of sequenced postures set to the rhythm of breath has been shown to be a much more recent development than many yogins have previously assumed.

One aspect of modern yoga that finds surprising continuity with ancient forms of Indian yoga and asceticism, however, is the use of material "props" to support one's yogic and meditative practice. In particular, the idea of using a cloth yoga strap or belt to fix one's body in a posture turns out to be at least two thousand years old![2]

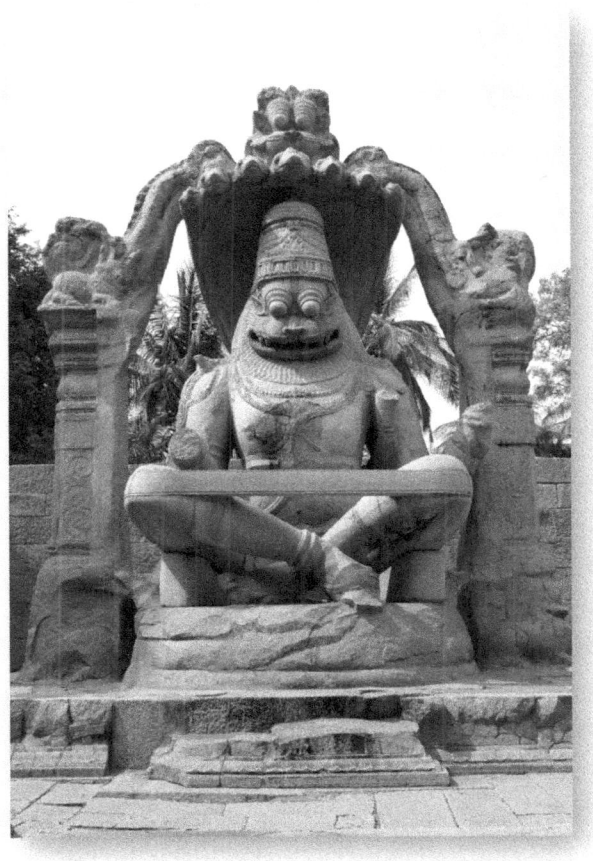

Yoga Narasimha *(half man, half lion), Hampi, Karnataka, India (c. 14ᵗʰ century).*
Photograph by Seth Powell.

In many ways, this use of a yoga prop is directly in alignment with the historical goal of asana, which was to prepare the body for sitting longer in meditation. Actually, the goal of yoga wasn't to just sit in meditation, but to transcend the body all together by reaching higher levels of consciousness known as *samadhi*, or enlightenment.

In these sculptures, the figures are sitting cross-legged with their knees raised and the strap is being used to support their legs and hips. It's placed around the lower back and then outside of the knees and tied tightly. The strap keeps the knees raised, which is less strenuous for the hips when sitting longer for meditation.

These days, asana has moved beyond just preparation for meditation and has become a science, even a sport, of its own. The real question is, what is the role of asana in yoga? If we can come to an agreement about that, then we can ask whether innovation and adaptation of asana is still in keeping with these overarching goals of the practice.

Unfortunately, it's very difficult to come to an agreement about the goals of yoga because these goals have changed greatly over the thousands of years that yoga has been practiced. Plus, yoga is such a dynamic and diverse practice that it has often been used by different lineages and teachers for very different reasons.

Some people still travel what is basically a monastic path toward self-realization, although I think it is rare these days to find a yoga practitioner who is also living as a monk, dedicating their lives to their spiritual evolution. Today, most yoga practitioners are householders who are practicing yoga as a way to reduce their suffering, and to live more fulfilling and healthier lives.

Regardless of which goal you choose for your practice; it seems that adapting asana is an essential part of yoga. You can adapt the practice to your body if you're working toward enlightenment just as well as you can adapt the practice to your body if you're simply looking to reduce anxiety and find moments of peace in your otherwise chaotic life.

The Role of Asana

One of the ways to respect the tradition of yoga is to educate yourself about its history and philosophy, understanding that it's an indigenous practice from South Asia shared generously with the world. Yoga philosophy focuses on calming the mind so that we can connect with our divine essence, and practicing service (*karma yoga*) by dedicating our lives and our actions to the benefit of all humanity. Teaching yoga is best approached as a form of service. In fact, with that intention teaching becomes a medium to connect, serve, and love your students.

The ancient yoga teachings speak very little about the physical practices, but there is a clear understanding that the body and the mind are essential vehicles for our spiritual journey, and that they should be taken care of in a thoughtful and yet neutral way. Asana provides a much more grounded approach to what are generally ethereal and esoteric concepts. That means yoga asana works whether you have a conscious spiritual practice or not.

Asana can be a moving meditation focusing on energy and breath as we flow through our physical practices. Asana can directly calm the nervous system and quiet the mind in a way that non-body-based practices, such as mindfulness, cannot. The popularity of yoga often rests on the profound efficacy of asana, offering a very physical and tangible way to work with the subtle nervous system and intangible mind.

To balance tradition and innovation in asana it's important to keep in mind these basic ideas about yoga's past and purpose: asana is not simply about your own physical health, your strength, or your flexibility. To practice asana in a respectful way means that we connect to the larger spiritual goals of this ancient tradition, either explicitly or implicitly. Having a reverent attitude and having a willingness to learn are the two most essential elements in cultivating a practice that honors the tradition.

When you innovate without regard for the historical lineages of yoga asana, you are more likely to appropriate a culture and practice that is not yours. Marketing a new brand or style of yoga is typically not in alignment with the tradition and is more rooted in capitalist commodification. Instead, the way forward is to innovate so that you can go deeper yourself, and so that you can share yoga more effectively with your students. As long as the innovation is based in service—which comes out of care and love, and oriented toward honoring the roots of yoga—then you are practicing in alignment with yoga's fundamental ethical teachings.

Adapting asana can also make yoga practice accessible to the most marginalized among us. Simplifying poses, practicing in a chair or in bed, can make the power of yoga available to a significant number of people who aren't interested in the athletic asana practice that is so popular these days. Making yoga accessible is directly aligned with yoga's spiritual essence. Yoga's most basic message is that we all share the same heart, and by creating ways for us to practice yoga together, we can experience the diversity of our humanity as we simultaneously discover the universality of our spiritual connection.

Sharing the Essence of Yoga with All

As I mentioned, in order to make yoga accessible, we first need to reflect deeply on what yoga is. On the surface it seems easy to answer, but it is such a good question to consider time and time again. The simplest answer is that yoga is union with the true Self—a union between the ego-mind and spirit. Of course, it's also useful to spend time reflecting on what we mean by spirit or Self. Maybe you prefer another word: Consciousness, divine essence, God, Higher Power. You can also use the Sanskrit terms *Atman* or *Purusha*.

The Yoga Sutras of Patanjali, book 1 sutra 2, states, "*yogas chitta vritti nirodhah*," or "restraint of the modifications of the mind-stuff

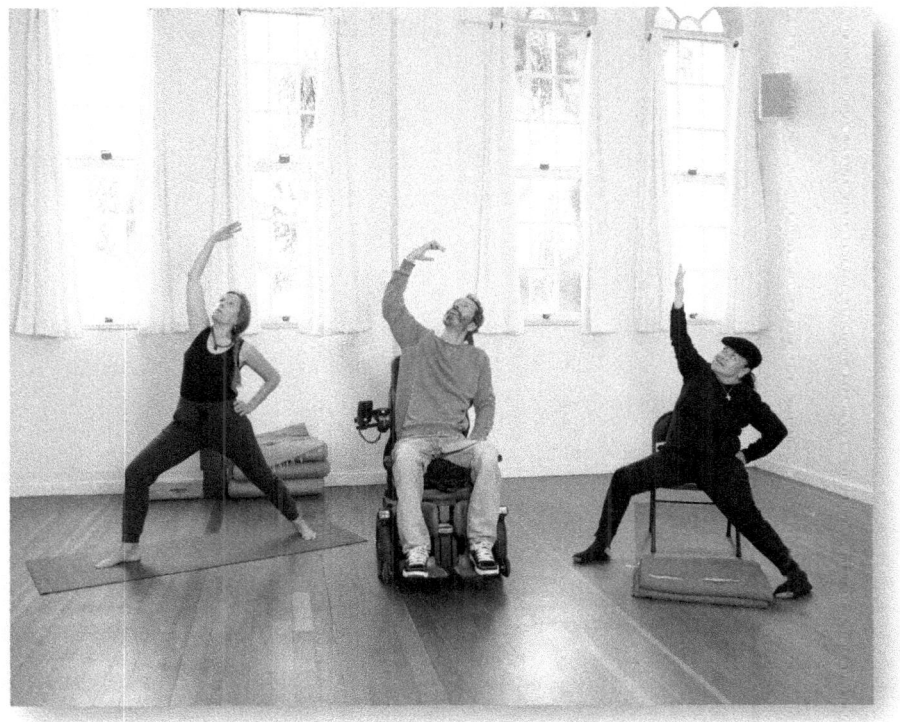

Three students practice in an integrated Accessible Yoga class. One student is standing on a mat, one is in a power wheelchair, and one is in a folding chair. They're all doing variations of reverse warrior pose, viparita virabhadrasana.

is yoga." Or, as I like to think of it, "peace of mind is yoga." Most of us have heard this sutra and considered its deep meaning, and yet it still holds mystery.

Generally speaking, we have identified with our mind, whether we have a spiritual bent or not. Even if we're immersed in spiritual practice, the mind usually retains its stronghold on our identity. But what if this basic assumption of who we are is wrong?

In the *Kena Upanishad*, there is a famous story of a fabled musk deer who spends its life searching for the source of an intoxicating musky fragrance. The deer searches far and wide, never finding the source of this intoxicating scent. It turns out that the musk deer has a gland that exudes this fragrant musk. Like a rabbit chasing a carrot on a stick, the deer is searching outside for something found within. Are we like the musk deer, ignorant of the source of our own happiness?

We see this same concept throughout the yoga teachings—the idea that what we seek is actually already within us, as us. Perhaps it is expressed most beautifully in this well-known quote from the *Chandogya Upanishad*, which is approximately 2,500 years old:

> *The little space within the heart is as great as this vast universe. The heavens and the earth are there, and the sun, and the moon, and the stars; fire and lightning and winds are there; and all that now is and all that is not: for the whole universe is in It and It dwells within our heart.*[3]

The yoga teachings and these spiritual concepts can be very subtle, and there may be moments where you grasp them and other times when they seem elusive. The mind can easily lull us into a state of dreamy ignorance where we don't bother diving deeper. It's important that we are all given the time and space to explore these concepts in a way that feels comfortable and safe for us. There is no timeline or agenda for spiritual exploration. Plus neither you nor your students have to agree with all the spiritual teachings of yoga, but you do need to understand them to the best of your ability.

Unfortunately, traumatic events and deep pain tend to bring these spiritual questions to the forefront. It's often in these challenging moments that we search for answers to life's eternal questions, "Who am I? Why am I here?" This is why challenging experiences can be such a powerful source of spiritual awakening, and often it's these challenges and suffering that bring us to yoga.

You may have come to yoga because of your own challenges, and now you wish to share what you discovered with others. But it's important that we avoid proselytizing, and that we give everyone space to find their own way, in their own time.

With this understanding, we also see that it's not our job to heal our students. Rather, we need to give students the tools to connect with and heal themselves at their own pace. With this understanding, we can release attachment to our success or failure and focus on service, or karma yoga. This is clearly expressed in the Bhagavad Gita, where Krishna explains to Arjuna that we can only find peace when we practice karma yoga by releasing attachment to our personal desires.

> *Someone with personal desires will not experience true peace. But when all desires merge, like different rivers flowing into the vast, deep ocean, then peace is easily realized.*[4]

What Is Accessible Yoga?

I'm always curious about the ways the term "Accessible Yoga" is understood and translated by the yoga community. What I've noticed recently is that some yoga teachers talk about making yoga accessible to their students in an effort to help them fit into their yoga classes—to help them conform.

Some teachers only offer different variations of a practice when a student can't do the "full expression" of a pose. In this case, the adapted practice is provided as some kind of consolation prize.

That's not exactly what I had in mind when I started teaching Accessible Yoga. My goal is, and has always been, to make the tools of yoga accessible to people in order to support them in personalizing the practice, so they can find an inner sanctuary. I remember one student saying that our class was like the Island of Misfit Toys, which was a sanctuary for all the rejected toys in the movie *Rudolph the Red-Nosed Reindeer*. I'm not sure how accurate that analogy was, but I appreciate the idea that we had created a space where anyone who felt they didn't belong was welcome and embraced.

While all yoga teachers need to know how to adapt the practice so that anybody can join their classes, that's really just the beginning. The ultimate goal is to celebrate our students' differences. This means actually celebrating the things that they may be ashamed of, and are hiding from the world. Can you imagine what it would be like to have your yoga teacher celebrate your differences? It would bring validation, a sense of being seen, and a feeling of belonging. It would lay the groundwork for transformational acts of self-acceptance and self-love.

The most fundamental teaching of yoga is that we are all inherently whole—*full*—and complete spiritual beings. Yoga begins with this positive assertion. You are already full. This assumption of our completeness is described in the Yoga Sutras of Patanjali. As I mentioned, Patanjali first defines yoga as the effort to calm the mind. Then he explains in sutra 1.3 that once the mind is calm, "The Self abides in its own true nature."[5] In other words, when the mind is peaceful, we automatically experience the truth of our spiritual essence. When the storm passes, we see that we're still standing.

In 1.4, he continues on to explain that when we're not abiding in our true nature, we're trapped in our thoughts. He says, "At other times, the Self assumes the form of the thoughts."[6] What he's describing is our fundamental human condition: We've forgotten the truth of our spiritual essence and, instead, identified with the thoughts in the mind. We've gotten lost and become disconnected from that place within our own heart. We've identified with our fleeting thoughts rather than with our immortal spirit.

The yoga practices are all designed to lead us back home to ourselves. They're not about giving us something new, or making us into something else. They're not about healing us, fixing us, or fitting us into a mold. But rather, peeling away the layers, like stripping away the layers of paint from wood furniture.

I have a background in art, and this idea of removing what's in the way, always reminds me of making a sculpture. There are two different traditional approaches to sculpture. In additive sculpture you build a sculpture from nothing. You use a medium like clay, and you build it up. You keep adding to it until it creates the image you have in your mind.

Another technique, called subtractive sculpture, is about carving and taking away. Usually the medium is stone or wood, and you actually take away that which is blocking the truth of the form. Great examples of this are Michelangelo's famous "non-finito" (unfinished) sculptures. These are giant male figures that seem to be coming out of the stone. It looks like they're emerging from the solid rock and transforming into something organic and alive.

In a famous quote, Michelangelo explained, "I saw the angel in the marble and carved until I set him free." That's the image that comes to mind when I think about Accessible Yoga. As teachers, we are supporting people as they reconnect with themselves—as they free themselves from the grasp of a culture that is always telling them they are not enough. We help them to discover and embrace their own fullness, and we show them that they can set themselves free.

Accessible Yoga is an approach to teaching based on the ideals of inclusivity, diversity and accessibility, rather than a specific style of yoga. It is defined by these concepts:

1. Everyone has a right to the teachings and practices of yoga
2. Each individual is a unique and equal expression of our universal connectedness
3. Service and compassion are yoga in action
4. Teaching yoga is a collaborative and creative process
5. Personal growth and transformation require a supportive community

What Does a Yoga Practitioner Look Like?

I saw a social media post the other day where someone was complaining about their yoga teacher including too many "other things" in their yoga class, such as talking about philosophy, chanting, breathing practices, and meditation. "Why can't you just teach yoga?" they exclaimed. Needless to say, this made my eyes roll because that is yoga! But then I stopped to think about it.

This person was expressing frustration based on what they believe to be true. Yoga has been portrayed in popular media as a purely physical practice for those who are agile, strong, and young. But this is finally shifting. More and more we're seeing a clearer representation of the truth of yoga—although we still have a long way to go!

One of the obstacles that I see is a lack of diversity among yoga teachers. There are many experienced practitioners who decide not to become teachers because they don't think they look like the image of a yoga practitioner that they have in their minds. These tend to be people with diverse backgrounds and body types, and if they did become teachers they would contribute to the diversification of the field. So in many ways, this oppressive media imagery creates its own vicious cycle.

I even know a number of yoga teachers who won't teach publicity because they don't think people will come to their classes merely based on how they look or because they can't do some of the poses. These are disabled teachers, teachers with larger bodies, queer and trans teachers, older teachers, etc. Yoga will only become diversified and welcoming when people can see themselves reflected in their teachers.

We've been soaking in a cultural belief system that is based on ableist ideas. This includes the idea that disabled people are less valuable than nondisabled people. Similarly, fat people,[7] people of color, and old people, are all somehow less valuable than an idealized young, thin, flexible white person. Ableism has been particularly pervasive in a yoga culture that has emphasized the physical aspect of a practice that is literally about transcending our body.

Like a weed that creeps into all corners of our garden, these ideas of ability, strength, flexibility, health, wellness, and even ideas around life and death itself have limited our understanding of yoga practice as something that is only for certain people. Related to this is the idea that disabled people need to be fixed through yoga. I would include here people who work with mental health challenges, some of whom are reclaiming the word "mad," just as people with larger bodies are reclaiming, "fat," and gay people have reclaimed, "queer."

The word "disabled" has also been reclaimed by a generation of people who perceive disability as a central part of their identity, rather than something to overcome. While everyone has the right to use whatever language they choose to identify themselves, it's also important to reflect on the language we share in general use, and in our yoga teaching.

Let's not use yoga to reinforce these ableist ideas, and be sure to teach in a way that reflects the truth of the teachings. Yoga is a spiritual practice focused on giving us perspective on the complex relationship between our body and spirit. In many ways, the goal of the practice is a discerning mind that is freed from the limitations of our individual desires and can reflect the profound interconnectedness of our shared humanity.

Imposter Syndrome

In order to teach what you love, you need to overcome some of the challenges of becoming a teacher. Personally I found that the biggest hurdle was overcoming my insecurities. I've struggled with shyness my whole life. I would never speak in school, and I dreaded having the teacher call on me. I think I was so concerned about what others thought about me that I was frozen with fear. The first few years that I was teaching yoga, I would panic before each class and arrive sweaty, blushing, voice quaking.

In the very first class I ever taught, I had a student who was crying in the front of the class the entire time, and I didn't know what to do. She came in, laid down on her mat, and began crying as soon as class started. I was so overwhelmed with remembering what to say that I just had to ignore her. She came up to me after class and thanked me for letting her have the space to cry. She said she just felt like she needed to be in a safe place with other people.

I'm so glad that worked out because I didn't know what else to do. I was overcome with what I would call imposter syndrome. I didn't feel like I was capable of or fit for the job of yoga teacher, and in many ways I wasn't. That's the thing about imposter syndrome, there is usually a kernel of truth to it. But the question that we're faced with is: How am I going to respond to that truth?

We can turn toward it, and recognize our limitations, or we can ignore those feelings, and allow the imposter syndrome to grow into a paralyzing monster within us. The choice is ours. Luckily, with an effective practice, we have the opportunity for honest reflection, *svadhyaya.*

The truth is, I was a brand new teacher, and in many ways I was an imposter because I didn't really know what I was doing. At the same time, I was being honest with my students and myself that I was new. Taking the seat of a teacher is a high calling. It means that I practice yoga's ethical values to the best of my ability. It doesn't mean that I have to be a perfect being, but it does mean that when I mess up, I'm honest about it.

The problem with imposter syndrome is that if it goes too far it can paralyze you. How do you ever become an experienced teacher if you don't allow yourself to be a new teacher? The way to become masterful at something is by learning from your mistakes, and being honest with yourself. If I'm teaching a class and I'm 100 percent satisfied with myself as a teacher how can I improve? If I can see where

I might have made an error, or how I could have done better, that inspires me to grow and learn so I can become a better teacher.

For me, the other kernel of truth in imposter syndrome is that yoga is a massive subject. Yoga has grown and evolved over thousands of years in endless threads and traditions. It's impossible to be an expert on all of yoga. Rather, you can focus on one part that is meaningful to you and useful for your students. You can also be honest about the things you don't know.

You also have to be aware of your positionality. If you're not of South Asian descent, then you need to consider your relationship to the teachings. If you're only using the teachings for profit and approaching yoga teaching just as a job, then you are appropriating an ancient indigenous practice that has already been, and is still very much being, colonized and abused by Westerners.

It's also important to acknowledge that the history and traditions of yoga are not without problems themselves. Not only has there been tremendous abuse, which we'll discuss later, but the way that caste is embedded in the yoga teachings is very problematic. The caste system made the teachings of yoga inaccessible to many, and our teaching today needs to be part of the effort to debrahmanize yoga, which is to remove caste from the way we teach and practice. I'll discuss this further on page 210.

So it's not surprising that we often feel like imposters when identifying ourselves as yoga teachers, regardless of our background or knowledge. In her words that opened this chapter, Indu Arora, who is one of the most knowledgeable yoga teachers I know, says that she still sees herself as primarily a student.

Like I said, there's a kernel of truth to imposter syndrome, and we can use this truth to learn and grow. In fact, it reminds me of the yoga teachings about ego. Patanjali describes ego as a case of mistaken identity. The body and mind have lay claim to the power of the spirit. He explains, "Egoism, *asmita*, is the identification, as it were, of the power of the Seer (*Purusha*) with that of the instrument of seeing [body-mind]."[8]

Taking the Seat of the Teacher with Humility

After teaching for almost thirty years, I can say that yoga is truly accessible to everyone—if the teacher has the skills to make it so. That's the thing. The responsibility is on you, the teacher, to find a way to share the practice that works for the person in front of you, and that is asking a lot.

I'll start by saying that I adore yoga teachers and trust that you are caring and service-oriented. You have a very high calling. You are tasked with sharing an ancient and powerful practice, as well as creating a welcoming and safe environment for all students who come to you. In a way, you need to prepare to be the teacher for everyone, even if you won't be in the end.

Cultivating safety is multifaceted and individual. What feels safe for one person will not feel safe for somebody else. But, there are some techniques that you can use to cultivate personal agency in your students and create a safer environment. I'll cover these techniques in detail in this book. They include trauma-sensitive teaching, avoiding pose hierarchy, offering a spectrum of practices for all levels, learning how to teach different levels at the same time, respecting the tradition, avoiding gendered language, and more. You also need to work within your scope of practice, and refer out to other professionals if something is beyond your training.

I discussed how to work with imposter syndrome, but I also want to discuss the other side—the danger of letting teaching go to your head. When you teach you become a conduit of these ancient teachings and the power of yoga will flow through you. If you're not careful you and your students may begin to equate that power with your own personal ego. You'll fall into the trap of ego that Patanjali so succinctly described.

This is where humility, as well as peer support come in. Other teachers can help keep you grounded. If you let your students put you up on a pedestal—which many will want to do—then you will be the one who falls off and gets hurt. Yoga has tremendous benefits for all of us, but in order to remain free from your students' expectations, be careful not to let them create a hagiography around you and be careful to not believe it yourself. The answer is to find a balanced approach, embracing the role of teacher as a servant leader.

I admit I have a recurring dream, really a nightmare, about teaching yoga. Usually, in the dream I'm teaching in a very public setting, like a mall or a park, and there are hundreds of people milling about. I'm trying to get people to listen to me but they won't. Instead, I'm yelling my instructions to try to get their attention as they continue to pass by without noticing. I'm sure someone will analyze that dream for me, but it's pretty obvious that I'm struggling with taking the seat of the teacher—even after all these years! So I really hope you'll be patient with yourself.

Yoga teachers' responsibilities include:

- Welcome everyone to the practice
- Keep people safe. This includes keeping students safe from each other
- Working within your scope of practice, and referring out when appropriate
- Not appropriating yoga, which means teaching as service
- Citing your sources and your teachers
- Practicing yoga ethics, particularly in relationship to your students
- Remaining a student always & committing to your practice
- Having peer support

Responsibilities of a Yoga Student

I often talk about the responsibilities that rest on the shoulders of yoga teachers, which I'm describing in detail in this book. It is also useful to consider the role of the student so that we can support them as well as possible. Understanding the role of a student can also support our ongoing learning. After all, to be a teacher is to be a student first.

As students, we need to have clear boundaries and understand that it's our body, our life, and our practice. The more we can be in touch with our needs, the more effective the experience will be. Being a docile, receptive vessel is not always the safest and most effective approach to learning. When yoga teachers attend any of my continuing education programs, I begin by telling them, "You don't need to arrive as a blank slate. Bring your whole self, and your life experience to everything that you do."

Rather than giving up our power to the teacher, we engage in a collaborative learning experience: It's a give-and-take. The teacher is making suggestions, and we are using those suggestions to inform our process.

As a student, it's useful to consider some of the following questions:

- What is my role in the learning process? Am I an empty cup, or does my past experience and knowledge impact how I learn?
- What is my favorite way to learn: visual, auditory, or kinesthetic?
- Knowing what my learning style is, what is the most effective environment or way for me to learn? Would I do best taking in-person classes, or online? Do I learn by listening to lectures or reading books?
- What are the goals of my practice? Am I looking for strength and flexibility, stress-reduction, spiritual awakening, something else?
- What qualities am I looking for in a yoga teacher?
- Do I understand consent and how to say no and when to stop?
- Can I respect the boundaries of the teacher and other students?
- Am I putting my yoga teacher up on a pedestal? Can I remember that they are human and not to be idolized?

- Do I understand my yoga teacher's scope of practice and find additional support when needed?

Reflection

What is your mission or goal as a yoga teacher? Can you write up an intention for yourself? The Accessible Yoga Teacher Promise below is my personal intention:

Accessible Yoga Teacher Promise

As an Accessible Yoga Teacher, I affirm the humanity and divinity of each individual who crosses my path, and I promise to share the yoga teachings with all who seek them. I will strive to make the practices of yoga accessible to all of my students regardless of ability or background, and to serve with love and compassion.

Scenario

A fellow trainee in the yoga teacher training that you're enrolled in comments on the fact that the training includes lots of adapted practices. They say something like, "I'm not interested in chair yoga, I'm planning to teach 'advanced,' students, so why do I need to learn all that?"

Response

Believe it or not, I've heard this kind of comment from many yoga teachers, and even some people in charge of major yoga organizations. I have a number of responses to this:

1. Even if you're not the teacher for everyone, you should train as if you could be. You never know who will be attracted to you and end up in your classes.
2. In the U.S. the ADA (Americans with Disability Act) states that reasonable accommodations need to be made so that all public offerings are accessible to people with disabilities.[9]
3. According to the Centers for Disease Control, 1 in 4 people in the U.S. identify as disabled[10], so chances are you have disabled students in your classes whether you know it or not.
4. Why would you limit yourself to only teaching non-disabled people? Don't you want to have a large number of students and expand your pool of potential students?
5. Older students, temporarily disabled students, students with larger bodies, and really all of us, can benefit from adapting practices.
6. Are you planning to practice and/or teach yoga as you get older?
7. Don't you think our teaching should be an expression of the yoga teachings themselves? How can we exclude anyone from practicing when the heart of yoga speaks to our universal connection?

Further Reflection

- Reflect on why you teach yoga and what yoga means to you.

- Find a way to express this clearly without prose-lytizing.

- Consider ways that you can teach yoga throughout your life. Try to be generous with the information you received. Share yoga with your family and friends. Talk about it openly and how it serves you including philosophy, subtle practices, and asana.

CHAPTER TWO

THESE GREAT VOWS: ETHICS FOR TEACHERS

When I first studied the yamas and niyamas, they were taught to me as proscriptive. "This is what you should do, or you shouldn't do. Avoid violence, and give up harming, and stealing, and lying, etc." But now, I actually look at them in a completely different way. I no longer view them as proscriptive. I see them as descriptive. They describe how an integrated person acts. In summary, an integrated person treats themselves and others with respect.

Considering that, I began to believe that teaching yoga is not a right, it is a privilege. When we remember that as teachers, it's very humbling. We get to spend our lives mirroring the inherent goodness and inner wisdom of our students. We have the privilege of offering them a way to shift their consciousness, which can hopefully make their lives and the lives of everyone they come in contact with a little better.

I'm even beginning to feel that there's another level to this. We have a responsibility because through our practice and training—through what we've learned, and what we've read, and what we've understood—we've been given the great gift of this practice, handed down from person to person for centuries.

As we mature as teachers, we have a responsibility to share our best selves with the world. It's our responsibility to pass the gift of yoga as clearly and as compassionately as we can. We have been given a treasure, now how are we going to share it?

The simplest way I can think of to describe ethics is related to the golden rule, treating others as we would like to be treated. We want to speak and act with that in mind when we take the seat of the teacher. We are opening ourselves to transmit this training, this particular lesson, these practices. First and foremost, these transmissions need to come from deep respect and compassion. How we touch our students. How we ask permission to touch. Where we touch. When we touch. When we decide not to touch. When do we ask our students to do something that's a little difficult for them? How do we do that in a way that recognizes their choice and power to say no, but also encourages them to take a small step forward into the sacred unknown of learning? Yoga is such a personal practice. It is the teacher and the student in a dance of respect and learning. That's how I like to think of ethics, and how I like to "practice" the yamas and niyamas while teaching yoga, as well as in my wider life.

—Judith Lasater

SEEING THE WHOLENESS of your students is essential. But, I'd suggest that the most important teachings of yoga that you need to consciously practice are the ethical teachings, the *yamas*. These days I think *brahmacharya* is particularly important in light of all the abuse that has happened in the yoga world over the last few decades.

Brahmacharya is traditionally translated as celibacy for monks, and these days it is interpreted as energy preservation, or awareness of how you are spending your energy. As a teacher, I like to think of it as focusing my energy on the yoga, and trying not to be distracted by all the things that surround it, such as notoriety, financial success, etc.

Almost every traditional lineage of yoga has had some history of abuse, and most are sexual in nature. So, it's essential that as a yoga teacher you spend time reflecting on your relationships with your students and consciously create healthy boundaries for them and for you. I think it's overly simplistic to say that you should not have relationships with your students, because in a way that's impossible. The student-teacher relationship is a valid relationship. It includes a kind of camaraderie that's essential in creating a supportive learning environment. The question is: How do you cultivate healthy student-teacher relationships based on mutual respect?

The way I approach it is to ask myself if I need anything from my students. Do I need their approval, their affection, or their friendship? If I feel like I'm being compensated fairly in other ways, then that is enough. This reflection is the key that has helped me to navigate my relationships with thousands of students over these many years. It starts by making sure I feel like I'm not being taken advantage of.

Part of this process is checking in with how you feel about the way you're pricing your offerings and making sure it feels fair. If you're a new teacher, then teaching for free might feel fine, but over time that feeling will probably change as you become more and more experienced.

Beyond payment, my goal is to try to get my personal needs met somewhere else, whether that is with my partner, my family, or my friends. I have had some friendships with students over the years, and I love them dearly. But as soon as I found myself needing something from them, then I knew I had crossed a boundary for myself, and I stopped considering them as students.

This approach, not trying to get my personal needs met from my students, is also a form of service, *seva*, or karma yoga. It's an effort to fulfill myself through my personal practice, rather than to constantly look for happiness outside. Unfortunately, service is a concept that is often misused by contemporary yoga culture to mean volunteering, and that's not the same thing. To be of service means to move from a place of love and care, rather than from a place of lack.

Part of the confusion comes from the students' tendency to conflate you and the teachings themselves. It's like drinking a cold glass of water when you are very thirsty. You feel grateful for the glass, after all it's harder to drink without it, but it's not the glass that's quenching your thirst. The teachings are like cool water, quenching our spiritual thirst. The vehicle for those teachings is admirable, but we shouldn't confuse the container for what's inside.

I always keep in mind that I didn't create these practices, and I am simply passing along what I was taught. Saying this aloud is important. In fact, acknowledging this at the beginning of a yoga class is a wonderful way to start. You can acknowledge your teachers, all those who have kept these practices alive for thousands of years, and offer gratitude for the teachings themselves.

Traditionally, yoga practice begins with guru mantras. These mantras express reverence and appreciation for the teacher and the teachings. In my tradition, we always started our meditation practice with this mantra:

Om namah Shivaya gurave
Satchidananda murtaye
Nishprapanchaaya shantaya
Niralambaya tejase

The Guru is auspiciousness
Embodiment of truth, knowledge, bliss
Salutations to the One beyond the worlds
Peaceful, independent and radiant.[11]

I think it's possible to find a way to bring in this traditional practice that is more aligned with a contemporary approach to the role of the teacher. Rather than thinking of the guru as an all knowing and all powerful external teacher, you can think of the concept of *guru tattva*, the guru principle, or the inner teacher that we all have within us. Or, you can think of the teachings themselves as the guru. After all, guru literally means the one who removes darkness, and it is the teachings themselves that hold that potential.

Non-Attachment

Generally, there is a lopsided power dynamic in the relationship between the teacher and the student, whether real or imagined. Often the student perceives themselves as having no power, and they perceive the teacher as having tremendous power. This is why romantic relationships between teachers and students are very challenging to navigate. If you start a relationship with one person having power and the other not, it can take a long time to shift away from that dynamic and create balance.

To truly embody the teachings as a yoga teacher means that you are working toward finding peace and fulfillment within yourself and within your practice, or at least you have a conscious awareness of your personal needs. The practice asks you to find, uncover, or reveal the truth that is always there hiding beneath your busy mind. To live that truth as a teacher means that you're independent and free from the need for external validation that might come from your students.

The problem is that the ego-mind loves to be stroked. It loves positive affirmation and all those compliments. It's a great practice to observe your mind's reaction to getting a compliment or not getting one. I still struggle with this personally, so I don't want to say it's easy. I love compliments, and I see how my mind often depends on them. But, what I'm working on is being kinder to myself, giving myself compliments, and no longer allowing my self-worth to be based on other people's opinions of me.

This is the practice of non-attachment, *vairagya*, which many people misconstrue as not having personal relationships or personal belongings. Non-attachment is really about understanding that my mind is colored by my personal beliefs and experiences. To be non-attached is to be neutral, to have clarity of vision, and to see beyond my personal wants and needs. Non-attachment allows me to perceive another person as a separate and yet equal being with their own complex inner world.

So the first step in becoming an effective yoga teacher isn't mastering teaching skills, but beginning to work with your own mind. At the very heart of the practice is non-attachment, the recognition that what you're seeking is with you. That practice can free you of any needs and expectations from your students, and allow you to have open, respectful, and effective teacher-student relationships. These are relationships with professional boundaries that offer your students the ultimate freedom to grow and flourish.

You Can't Have Spirituality Without Ethics

In 1990, when I was twenty-three, I had the luck of rediscovering yoga. My grandmother had taught me yoga when I was a young child, but I hadn't practiced again until life pushed me to. Thank God I did find it again, because it was a very painful time for me. I was a gay man living through the AIDS crisis. My friends were sick and dying. The grief was overwhelming, and I was completely falling apart.

Yoga helped put me back together. Not only did I find strength and relaxation, but I found comfort in the spiritual teachings at the core of the practice. Mostly, I found solace in the concept of the true Self, Purusha, living on past the death of our body and mind. That understanding of how part of us lives on helped me deal with so much loss at such a young age.

Previously, I had always rejected spiritual teachings because they were usually shrouded in homophobia. So much spirituality is connected to organized religion which excludes me as a queer person. Yoga felt different. The clarity, accessibility, and expansiveness of the teachings felt inviting. More than that, I could actually experience huge shifts in my body and mind through the practices. Asana, pranayama, and meditation provided an embodied spirituality that I had never experienced before. Yoga somehow circumvented my doubting mind and touched my broken heart.

Part of the power I was experiencing came from finding a strong spiritual community, a *sangha*. I felt grateful to have supportive friends and welcoming teachers at Integral Yoga, where I studied, taught, and eventually worked for decades. I felt especially lucky to have found a living guru in my teacher, Swami Satchidananda. But, at the same time, there were already accusations of him sexually abusing his students. A small group of women were speaking up. They even had a public demonstration in front of a venue where Swami Satchidananda was teaching in 1991. That protest may have been the very first public accusation of abuse by a yoga teacher in the U.S.[2]

When I asked senior teachers in our lineage what had happened, I was told that these women were "crazy," and that I should ignore them because he would never do that. In what is one of the biggest regrets of my life, I chose to believe the gaslighting, and continued to get more and more involved in the organization. I got so involved that I became an Integral Yoga Minister and was on the Integral Yoga Teachers Council, which was one of the main governing bodies of the organization.

Then about ten years ago, as the #MeToo movement was in full swing, I realized that I was being lied to. I believed those women, and I needed to speak up, which I started to do. I spent a number of years working within Integral Yoga trying to get them to address the abuse, but there was a complete blockade.

It was clear that I could no longer be part of an organization that knowingly lies about past abuse, and in doing so, fosters an environment for future abuse and continued harm. More than that, I realized that many of my teachers, who I learned so much from, weren't practicing the most basic and essential element of yoga—ethics. It was heartbreaking to realize that the very people who I looked up to—who had supported me, trained me, and cared for me—were in fact perpetuating harm.

I also began to see that living ethically isn't comfortable. It often means sacrificing the easy for the good, and I paid the price. Once I started to speak publicly about the abuse, I was shunned by the organization. I lost work and friends, but in the end I know it was the right thing to do.

Yama Comes First

Spirituality can be a confusing concept, and over the years I've seen how that confusion is often used to control people within spiritual communities. In fact, if you look at the history of abuse within yoga traditions, and throughout many religions, you can see the way that spirituality has been used as a foil for abuse.

Loyalty to the teacher is used as a mask for hiding abuse. Senior teachers in these organizations, who have devoted their lives to the abusive teacher, are often incapable of clearly seeing what's in front of them. Sometimes it's willful ignorance. Their power comes through their position of authority, and they may be unwilling to let it go. In doing so, they betray the very practices that they are attempting to uphold.

Personally, I find this to be one of the greatest ironies in life: Teachings and belief systems that are about freedom and overcoming suffering, are instead used to control, manipulate, and abuse. Spirituality can offer a sanctuary and a refuge from the challenges of life, but only if ethics are firmly established at its core. In fact, without ethics there is no spirituality.

In the yoga teachings, we see that the first limb of the classical eight limb path of *ashtanga* yoga is *yama*. These are the ethical teachings that we need to abide by in order to begin down the road of becoming a yoga practitioner. Yama includes *ahimsa* (non-harm), *satya* (truthfulness), *asteya* (non-stealing), *brahmacharya* (continence), and *aparigraha* (non-greed)—five relatively simple and straightforward ideas that are potent seeds for growing a healthy spiritual practice.

You can do all the fancy poses that you want, and sit in meditation for hours on end, but if you're not trying to live ethically, you're not doing spiritual practice. That is because ethics define the way we interact with other people, and even ourselves.

Most people think of spirituality as an inner journey, which is true. We need to treat ourselves ethically. But in so many ways, spirituality is about living in the world in a way that reflects the understanding that everything is spirit. This includes other people, animals, and nature. The way we treat others, and the world around us, is how our spiritual *practice* is put into action.

This is the challenge that so many of us face within traditional yoga lineages like Integral Yoga, Ashtanga Yoga, Sivananda Yoga Vedanta, and 3HO Kundalini. My teacher, Swami Satchidananda, was a powerful teacher, but he sexually abused his students. That abuse and lack of ethics makes me question the validity of all his teachings, which is incredibly confusing after having spent decades as his student. It leaves me with so many questions, and few answers.

How do I perceive him now? What about all the amazing things he taught me? Can I still consider him my teacher? How can I acknowledge my connection to a lineage, and to the South Asian roots of the practice, without acknowledging him?

After spending many years reflecting on this, I am starting to get some clarity. I see that Swami Satchidananda had access to a powerful wisdom tradition that existed beyond his individuality. These teachings are thousands of years old and have passed through many, many people.

I am incredibly grateful for what he taught me, but my devotion is no longer to him. My devotion is to the teachings themselves. Perhaps his greatest lesson for me was in his failure. In doing so he showed me the power of ethics. I now see that without ethics there is no yoga, and it gives me hope for myself and for our entire generation of yoga practitioners. We don't need to be perfect human specimens—but we do need to be ethical.

Ethics Create Accessibility

I teach people how to adapt practices. I can show you ten different ways to do a tree pose in a chair, or how to make pranayama trauma-informed. I enjoy the creativity and collaboration that goes along with this work. I love the idea of creating equity within yoga spaces, and how we can shift the dynamic within yoga classes to share power with our students. Adapting the practices for individuals has been an endless source of inspiration as well as challenge.

I love the universal nature of these teachings—the concept that we all share the same heart even though our lived experiences are completely different. That's why I've always said that if it's not accessible it's not yoga. But, what I've only recently realized, is that accessibility naturally flows from ethics. If I'm abiding by ethical teachings such as ahimsa, my number one priority is to make sure that I am not causing any harm. On the most basic level that means making sure that I'm not excluding anyone from the practice, and that I'm not hurting my students.

Obviously, I want to avoid abuse, whether it's physical, sexual, or emotional. But what about the subtle messages I may be sending? Can I be causing harm in other ways? Am I creating an environment that is toxic? This could look like expecting students to perform for me, or pushing them beyond their capacity. There could be even more subtle messages that are unspoken around who is invited to practice with me? Who is excluded?

If my teaching is not centered on accessibility and creating equity within yoga spaces, then I'm upholding harmful norms around appearance, performance, and ableism. The fact is, ethics provide a touchstone to connect back with when we're in the midst of life. As a yoga teacher, my job is to prioritize not causing harm, and to consider the many possible ways that may occur. This begins with deep inner reflection on the ways that I hold power, my social position, and how I might be upholding harmful systems.

Racism, in particular, has a way of seeping into yoga spaces, just as it enters into all public life. If you're a white, or white-presenting person, it's essential to educate yourself about racism and the ways that you may unknowingly be perpetuating harm. This could be through microaggressions, which are, "Brief and commonplace verbal, behavioral, or environmental indignities."[13] To learn more about anti-racism in yoga, I recommend the work of Michelle Cassandra Johnson, who is a contributor to this book.

Loving Kindness as an Ethical Practice

We usually define ahimsa as not harming, but a synonym for not harming is caring—and even loving. In many ways, the practice of ahimsa is the act of loving kindness. To love yourself and others is the goal of spirituality. It's that simple.

It's also essential to consider the role of satya, truthfulness. Honesty is the heart of integrity. It's a way to work with your own ego and selfishness. We often lie to protect ourselves, whether it's protecting ourselves from actual harm or just to protect the image that we are trying to project into the world. To be honest is to be utterly vulnerable. In that vulnerability we share the most tender part of our heart with ourselves and with others.

The question is, how do you practice ahimsa and satya in the role of yoga teacher? For starters, to avoid harm, you would make sure everyone felt welcome in your classes, and that would mean a lot. You would also teach in a way that focuses on sharing power with your students, so they have agency over their own body and their own experience. Most importantly, you would be honest about the challenges you face in your own practice, and have compassion for those who are struggling.

Individually, ahimsa and satya have the power to change lives. But combined, they create an explosive combination that can blast through even the most hardened heart. And that's the challenge: To be willing to feel deeply. Ethics isn't just about behaving in a righteous manner, it's also about being honest with your own feelings and your own suffering.

It reminds me of the character, Ebenezer Scrooge, from the 1843 book, *A Christmas Carol*, by Charles Dickens. Do you remember that classic story? After living a miserly life, Scrooge is visited by the ghosts of Christmas past, present, and future to show him a different perspective on his reality. In the end, his transformation hinges on experiencing the pain of his own life—by being honest with himself. From that truth, he was then able to feel the pain of others, and his newfound compassion transformed his life and the lives of those around him.

This is my prayer for all of us. Let us open our hearts to ourselves and to our own suffering, and allow that self-compassion to expand outward like a wave rippling in the ocean. The yoga practices are there to give us the strength to suffer consciously. In fact, that's how we avoid future suffering. When we practice, we gain an inner resilience by connecting to a deep place within us that is solid and unwavering.

These Great Vows

Patanjali makes many bold statements about ethics in the Yoga Su-tras. But in what may be his strongest statement in the entire book, after listing the five aspects of *yama*, in sutra 2.31 he exclaims, "These Great Vows are universal, not limited by class, place, time or circum-stance."[14] It's a bold claim. These are universal vows for all spiritual practitioners for all time.

Ironically, that translation of sutra 2.31 is by Swami Satchidan-anda, who I just talked about. So even as I share the power of ethics, I'm reminded of how challenging it is to practice them. I think the danger lies in expecting perfection rather than remembering that we are human and this is a practice. I know that I make mistakes and hurt people, usually by accident. Sometimes I twist the truth to make my ego-mind feel better. But as a practice, I try to reflect on why.

Eventually, I remember that causing harm and being untruthful only perpetuates my own suffering and ignorance. These great vows aren't there to punish us, but to set us free. The way out of suffering is through increased self-awareness. Every time I make a mistake and cause harm or lie, I can learn about the nature of my ego-mind. I can see the veil more clearly. Someday, with any luck, I'll actually be able to see through the veil and glimpse the truth of my inner light. When I do, I know it will be because I've been practicing ethics.

Reflection

What is your personal code of ethics? How do you practice the yamas in your relationships with your students?

- *Ahimsa*—what happens when a student says you have harmed them in some way? How do you respond?

- *Satya*—are you clear about your policies and do you stick to them when under pressure?
- *Asteya*—do you cite your sources and refer out to other professionals when needed?
- *Brahmacharya*—do you have healthy relationship boundaries with your students?
- *Aparigraha*—do you have expectations around your students' behavior? Are you relying on them for external validation?

Boundaries as Ethics

Usually we think of ethics as rules to follow. They seem like these external guardrails to control or limit our actions in some way. That may be partially true, but the way ethics are presented in yoga is much more of an internal guidance, like a GPS or a map to keep us from getting hurt and to lead us to peace. They're more like the bumpers in a bowling alley, which keep your ball from falling into the gutter. They help to keep you on track.

Ethics offer us protection. This is so important when you step into the role of teacher. You'll need to find clear, concise ways of protecting yourself and holding strong boundaries, not only for the sake of your students, but primarily for yourself. Without boundaries you may allow yourself to be used by your students, and through transference, they may act out their own internal dramas with you as a central character.

I remember one time I was teaching an ongoing class in a hospital conference room, and for some reason that day our class was moved into a much smaller room than usual. Of course, more people came that day, so the class was packed. The strange part was that same day one of my longtime students brought me a bouquet of flowers to thank me for my teaching. That went right to my head! I thought, "Wow, I must be really good at this."

But then as students kept coming, I had to ask the group to rearrange themselves a number of times. It was a very messy situation and kept delaying the start of the class. So finally, after a long, frustrating effort to fit everyone in the room, the same student who had brought me flowers stood up in the middle of the room and yelled at me, "You have no idea what you're doing, do you?"

In reflection, it was a funny moment that reminded me to not let things go to my head. Within a few minutes, this same student had both praised and criticized my teaching. It made me realize that I'm neither a great teacher nor a terrible one. I'm just doing my best.

Boundaries are the way we can protect our energy and our time. For example, an important boundary is not taking on your students' problems. Often students will come to you after class and ask for your advice. First, make sure you're speaking within your scope of practice, and second, don't allow yourself to become their personal support system. Of course, your class can be an important source of support for them. But once class is over, it's not okay for students to demand endless amounts of your time, or expect you to solve all their problems. If a student is struggling, you can refer them to a therapist or another service provider who is better suited to solve their problems.

It's often the most generous and caring teachers who don't have strong enough boundaries. They want to help everyone, and heal everyone. But usually, they end up suffering themselves. Don't allow that to happen to you. Know that by caring for yourself with strong and effective boundaries you can actually be more helpful to more people. Service starts at home. Care for yourself, your time, and your energy so that you can continue to teach for many years to come.

I remember one time when I didn't have healthy boundaries and paid the price. I had a longtime student with multiple sclerosis. She came to my weekly classes at a local community center, and would always transfer to the floor by herself even though some other students stayed in their chairs for the entire class. One day, she told me she hadn't been feeling well, and was experiencing extreme fatigue. It occurred to me that she would do well to stay in a chair that day. But instead of stepping in and saying something, I let her transfer to the floor, and practice the entire class that way.

At the end of class, as the other students were leaving, she said to me, "I can't get back up." So I proceeded to try to teach her a few techniques for getting up off the floor, and I knew a lot of them, but none of them worked. She was stuck on the floor, and since it was the end of the day there was literally no one around to help us. Without thinking it through, I proceeded to lift her up into a chair, and as I did so, I pulled a muscle in my back. It took me weeks to recover from that injury, and I realized that what I should have done is call emergency services to assist her, rather than take the situation into my own hands.

Scope of Practice for Yoga Teachers

Scope of practice is a legal term used mostly in medical professions, but it also applies to us as yoga teachers and yoga therapists. Scope of practice is basically the area that you're trained to work in. For example, if you're a medical doctor, you're trained to diagnose and treat patients regarding their physical health. If you're a psychologist, you're trained to address the needs of the mind. It is considered unethical to work outside of your scope of practice. Instead, you should refer your student or client to the appropriate professional given their needs.

For your reference, I wanted to include a brief discussion of the scope of practice of a yoga teacher as well as a yoga therapist. It was only a few years ago that Yoga Alliance came up with an official scope of practice for yoga teachers, which consists of six points:

1. Follow the Yoga Alliance™ Code of Conduct
2. Teach yoga
3. Adjust posture or practice with explicit and informed consent
4. Share yogic philosophy, history, and anatomy
5. Advise and teach within permitted scope
6. Maintain relevant credentials[15]

I think they should have added a point about adapting yoga practice or making it accessible to all your students, but they do at least refer to their Code of Conduct, which does speak to those points in detail. In fact, I was involved in the committees that helped shape the Code of Conduct, and I think it is a very useful document. It's too long to include here, so I would encourage you to read it on their website, even if you're not interested in participating in Yoga Alliance.

Scope of Practice for Yoga Therapists

Yoga therapy is still a relatively new profession, at least in its current form. The main governing body for yoga therapists is the International Association of Yoga Therapists (IAYT). I was a member when they created their educational standards in 2014, and I was involved in some of the conversations about those standards, including conversations about creating their scope of practice guidelines. It's too detailed to include the entire document here, but I encourage you to go to IAYT's website to read it.

I would like to highlight a few points which differentiate yoga therapy from yoga teaching, which I'm paraphrasing below. The following are considered to be within a yoga therapist's scope of practice:

1. Conduct a detailed assessment
2. Collect and store medical information

3. Develop a therapeutic plan that includes client's goals
4. Provide follow up and homework to cultivate client's personal practice
5. Interact with client's healthcare team[16]

In particular, yoga therapists are trained to handle confidential medical information, and yoga teachers are not. So, as a yoga teacher, it's important to be careful about what questions you ask your students. For example, rather than asking if they have medical issues they would like to share with you, you could simply ask if there is anything they want to share with you that would help you keep them safe during the practice.

Scenario

A student asks, "Do you want to go get some coffee after class?"

Response

When it comes to ethical questions for yoga teachers, I like to look at three elements. What can I do before, during, and after the interaction to support my ability to act ethically? Regarding this situation, it's actually more complicated than it may seem. On the one hand, a student asking you out for coffee may be a completely innocent and friendly gesture. But, it's important to have firm boundaries to protect yourself and your students.

On a professional level, the way to think about boundaries is to consider your scope of practice, which I mentioned above. Your scope of practice will actually protect you in the end, and I don't just mean protect you legally, although it may do that also. If the student is asking you out so they can discuss their life and their problems with you in detail, they might be asking you to act outside of your scope by expecting you to be their counselor or therapist.

Being friends with students isn't the problem, and as I mentioned earlier, I know that in some communities it's helpful when the teacher socializes with the students. The issue comes when the students start having expectations of you outside of class. Previously, I discussed ways to keep strong boundaries with your students, and I would encourage you to reflect on that.

It's especially important to find ways to do this in a friendly manner that doesn't feel cold or offensive. This is where having preset guidelines can be helpful. For example, you could have some simple policies on your website or intake forms which talk about how important ethics and professionalism are for you. Then when a situation like this arises you could say something like. "That's so kind of you to ask, and I appreciate that you want to spend time with me. I have a policy of not socializing with my students, but I encourage you to connect with the other students."

Further Reflection

- Can you practice ahimsa toward yourself? How?

- How can healthy boundaries with your students support you in your teaching and support them in their learning?

- Reflect on why there has been so much abuse in the yoga community, and commit to addressing it to the best of your ability.

- Reflect on your scope of practice. What specifically are you trained to teach your students?

CHAPTER THREE

BEYOND THE EIGHT
LIMBS OF YOGA

What I love so much about yoga is that there's something in there to address whatever we're going through, and different things hit at different times. And right now, what's hitting me is the teaching that we are all already whole. In this society, we're not encouraged to believe in our inherent wholeness. We're constantly looking for fulfillment in things that are outside of us.

We think that if we find the right person, then we'll be whole. If we have the house, then we'll be whole. If we have the kids, then we'll be whole. And the world feeds on that. It's constantly telling us, "If you buy this thing, you're going to be whole. Join this group, you're going to be whole." And yoga is like, "You are already whole. You don't believe it, because of all the stories, and the trauma, and all the messages that you've picked up throughout your life. But you were born whole, equipped with everything you need to thrive, honestly, as a human being on this planet."

If we lean into that wholeness, we can instead make yoga a destruction process, or really a taking-away process—a dismantling process. A lot of people talk about Shiva being about destruction, but what does that mean? He's also called the Adiyogi, which means "the first yogi" as well. So what does that mean? It means that yoga is a destruction process. It's taking away all that stuff that we've picked up and thought was us, and that we've just hung on to, and dismantling that.

That's the destruction that comes with the knowledge of yoga. So then what are we left with? We're left with wholeness, utter wholeness, full and complete. This is a message of yoga that I have to lean into these days, because it's hard to believe that I'm okay. But yoga reminds me that I've got everything I need. I am equipped. Doesn't matter what comes into my life. I can handle it. Right? When the world is telling me, "You need to do this. You got to do this. You got to do that." No, I'm full. I am whole. Let me sit in that, and go beyond the voices that are telling me that I am not.

—**Shanna Small**

YOGA IS A PRACTICE of spiritual awakening. This is one theme that we see clearly in all yoga traditions and texts. As much as we think of yoga as a primarily physical practice, all the texts I've studied state clearly that spiritual awakening is the goal. It's not so much about becoming something as clearing up our perception of ourselves. We are spiritual beings, and our work, or practice, is to remove the obstacles in the way of our experience of this essential nature.

We are born full and whole. That's the starting point, the foundation, the beginning and the end of our practice. We don't need to achieve or get something, we just need to recognize this fullness that already exists in us, as us. This is expressed beautifully in the *Brihadaranyaka Upanishad*, which is about three thousand years old:

Om purnam adah purnam idam
purnat purnam udachyate
purnasya purnam adaya
purnam evavasisyate

That is full this also is full.
This Fullness came from that Fullness.
Though this Fullness came from that Fullness
That Fullness remains forever full.
Om peace, peace, peace.[17]

In the Yoga Sutras, Patanjali shares a dualistic philosophy and asks us to differentiate between what is spirit, Purusha, and what is creation, *prakriti*. In fact, much of his philosophy is about separating these two elements—unyoking them. This always gets my attention, because we usually talk about yoga as union, and in many ways, Patanjali is presenting a case for yoga as separation. In particular, separation from identification with the body and mind. This is why I was so excited when Shanna Small shared this idea of yoga as a path of destruction, or clearing away.

The destruction that comes from yoga doesn't have to be monumental. It can be a small opening, or window of opportunity. Often these openings come when we are struggling or feeling challenged in some way. These shifts are where the power of yoga really shines. In many ways, yoga is magic, but not in the way we think. The magic of yoga comes from the slightest deepening of awareness, by the smallest shift in consciousness. This is a shift from doing to being—from identifying with the thoughts to observing them.

Do you talk to yourself in your mind? Are you narrating your own life? Do you ever wonder what part of you is talking, and what part is listening? The magic of yoga comes from identifying with the spirit, witness, or listener, instead of the mind talking.

Reflection

Who is talking in your mind?

Four Essential Yoga Texts

In a well-intentioned effort to move beyond the limits of modern yoga's obsession with asana, a lot of teachers talk about practicing all eight limbs of yoga. I'm always grateful to see this expansion of our focus beyond the physical. The thing is, there's a lot more to yoga than just eight limbs.

It can be helpful to study source texts directly, including the Yoga Sutras of Patanjali, where the eight limbs are found. Other important texts include the Bhagavad Gita, the Upanishads, and the *Hatha Yoga Pradipika*.

My sense is that as yoga continues to expand, more and more texts will be translated into different languages and become more broadly available. We'll also be exposed to texts written in languages other than Sanskrit. One example of this is the *Kural* by Tiruvalluvar, which is a Tamil text that is just as old as the Upanishads. The *Kural* is a powerful reflection on how to live a happy life, with an emphasis on ethics. What is also remarkable about this text is that it contains deep spiritual teachings right alongside practical lessons for daily life. One of my favorite quotes is about non-attachment and how we can find freedom by attaching to spirit:

> *Cling to the One who clings to nothing;*
> *And so clinging, cease to cling.*[18]

Upanishads

The Upanishads are a group of texts that date broadly from 800 BCE to 500 CE, and form the heart of *Sanatana dharma*, the eternal path. The early Upanishads are the ones that are most well-known and most frequently studied. Collectively they are referred to as Vedanta (meaning the end of the Vedas), and offer a straightforward discourse on spirituality.

The term "upanishad" literally means to sit down near a teacher[19] and reflects the conversational format of these texts. Often these are dialogues between teacher and student, or in the case of the *Brihadaranyaka Upanishad*, a conversation between husband and wife. There is a famous quote from this text that speaks to the pursuit of spiritual realization by renouncing the natural world and transcending selfish desire.

> *You are what your deep, driving desire is.*
> *As your desire is, so is your will.*
> *As your will is, so is your deed.*
> *As your deed is, so is your destiny.*[20]

This is the kind of timeless truth revealed in the Upanishads. Questions of desire, will, destiny and spirituality found in engaging dialogues. From the perspective of the ego-mind, we usually think of ourselves as humans trying to have a spiritual experience. The Upanishads ask us to turn that around and consider ourselves spiritual beings having a temporary human experience. Could that be the essence of yoga: this shift in perspective so small, and yet so powerful?

This new perspective is a uniquely positive one: We are spirit, and though our mind and body are limited by space and time, we are not. The result of this shift is that we realize we are the source of our own joy, and we have what we need within. This shift in identification can come from deep practice or spontaneous realization. According to the *Katha Upanishad*:

> *There are two selves, the separate ego*
> *And the indivisible Atman. When*
> *One rises above the 'I' and 'me' and 'mine,'*
> *The Atman is revealed as one's real Self.*[21]

The *Isha Upanishad*, is often considered to be one of the oldest and most important Upanishads. It is a brief and powerful celebration of universal spirit, and urges us to uncover that spirit in our lives. One compelling verse speaks to the idea of seeing yourself in others, which has been at the heart of my teaching and a core aspect of Accessible Yoga:

> *Those who see all creatures in themselves*
> *And themselves in all creatures know no fear.*
> *Those who see all creatures in themselves*
> *And themselves in all creatures know no grief.*
> *How can the multiplicity of life*
> *Delude the one who sees its unity?*[22]

The Upanishads greatly influence later texts such as the Bhagavad Gita and the Yoga Sutras of Patanjali, and are the original source for many yoga teachings that we continue to use today. For example, the concept of the *panchamaya kosha*, the layers of being, comes from the *Taittiriya Upanishad*.

Bhagavad Gita

The Bhagavad Gita is a sacred text from India that dates back approximately three thousand years. Within the Gita, whose title means "The Song of the Divine," are some of the most essential yoga teachings presented in a very accessible format. Similar to the Yoga Sutras of Patanjali, the Bhagavad Gita defines yoga as calming the mind:

> *Equanimity of mind is yoga. Do everything, Arjuna, centered*
> *in that equanimity. Renouncing all attachments, you'll enjoy*
> *an undisturbed mind in success or failure.*[23]

The entire Gita is an allegory for the difficult battle we all face in subduing our selfishness and attachment to the material world. Krishna teaches Arjuna that the true Self is eternal and unchanging, and that to know that Self, we must conquer our selfishness and ego. Similar to themes in the Upanishads, the Gita teaches that it is this inner battle that defines a yogi as one who has identified with spirit instead of mind. Through this connection with the Self, we also overcome pain and sorrow, leading to a peaceful and blissful life.

Yoga is a means to disconnect your identification with that which experiences pain. Therefore, be determined to steadily practice yoga with a one-pointed mind.

Completely let go of all personal desires and expectations. Then with your own mind, you can withdraw the senses from all sides. Little by little your mind becomes one-pointed and still, and you can focus on the Self without thinking of anything else.

However your mind may wander away, continue to draw it back again to rest in the true Self.

The one who has trained the mind to stay centered in equanimity, in this life, has cast aside both good and evil karma. Therefore, by all means practice yoga; perfection in action is yoga.[24]

Krishna explains that through wisdom, devotion, meditation, and service, we can overcome the powerful ego, and experience the divinity within. His teachings can be summarized as the four traditional paths of yoga, which give a hint to the expansiveness of this practice. These four paths are: *jnana yoga*, the path of wisdom; *bhakti yoga*, the path of devotion; *karma yoga*, the path of action and service; and *raja yoga*, the path of concentration and meditation.

Jnana yoga:

> *If your mind is unsteady and wandering, many-branched and endless are the thoughts and choices. When your mind is clear and one-pointed, there is only one decision.*[25]

Bhakti yoga:

> *I love that devotee who maintains equanimity during praise and blame; who takes refuge in silence (wherever they may be); who is content (no matter what occurs); whose home is every-where; whose mind is always steady; and whose heart is full of devotion.*[26]

Karma yoga:

> *The ignorant work for their own profit, Arjuna; the wise work for the welfare of the world, without thought for themselves.*[27]

Raja yoga:

> *The well-trained mind of a yogi, concentrating on the Self, is as steady as a flame in a windless place.*[28]

Hatha Yoga Pradipika

These main early philosophical texts of yoga barely discuss the physical practices of yoga, known collectively as *hatha yoga*. In fact, there are only three sutras in the Yoga Sutras of Patanjali that directly address the topic of asana. On the other hand, we do find depictions of yogis practicing asana in early sculpture, as I discussed in chapter one. There are also later texts that discuss the physical practices in detail. The most well-known of these is the *Hatha Yoga Pradipika*, which was composed by Svatmarama in the 1400s.

Svatmarama was believed to be part of the lineage of Nath yogis, which was a very important tradition of yoga based on devotion to the god Shiva. The lineage also includes Matsyendranath, for whom the seated spinal twist is named.

The *Hatha Yoga Pradipika* includes fifteen detailed asana practices, but is primarily concerned with *prana*, life force or subtle energy, and the ways we can learn to work with it. These include *pranayama*, breathing practices; *mudra*, energy seals; and *bandha*, energy locks. The text explores many esoteric practices. Most are in common usage today, but there are others that are extremely complicated and potentially dangerous.

The *Pradipika* is an interesting example of how much things have changed over the last six hundred years—and how some things haven't changed at all! He is speaking to a true yogi, a person who has dedicated their entire life to yoga and to their spiritual journey. This is most likely a *sannyasin*, a monk, who has released many of their ties to the world. They probably have taken vows of celibacy, poverty, and non-attachment. This is also why you should use the term "yogi" or "yogini" with care and consider that even though you may be a dedicated yoga practitioner, you are probably not a yogi in this traditional sense of the word.

This complete dedication to a somewhat ascetic practice is so different from the yoga practice we see in common usage today. Yoga today is often used to promote physical healing and wellness, fitness, and even physical beauty. Svatmarama's spiritual teachings are clearly at odds with a contemporary practice that focuses on external achievement and attachments. Instead, he is teaching us to use the body as a vehicle for spiritual attainment.

What feels like it hasn't changed in six hundred years, is the heart of the practice that is still alive in so many dedicated practitioners around the world. This is the effort to transcend our limited ego-mind and connect with our true Self. Plus, so many of the practices Svatmarama shares are very much a part of yoga practice today, such as forward bends, peacock, twist, bow, lion, *viparita karani mudra, shavasana, ujjayi, nadi shuddhi, kapalabhati*, and many more.

Chapter one deals with setting the proper environment for yoga, the ethical duties of a yogi, and the asanas. Fifteen poses are described, and seven of them are seated postures, which speaks to the emphasis on asana being preparation for subtler practices—most of which are done seated.

> *Hatha yoga is a sheltering monastery for those scorched by all the [three] kinds of suffering. Hatha yoga is a foundational support for those who are engaged in the practice of different kinds of yoga. (Three kinds of suffering are those arising from natural causes, other living beings, and oneself.)* [29]

> *One who practices hatha yoga should live alone in a small monastery, situated a bow's length away from rocks, water, and fire, in a virtuous, well-ruled kingdom which is prosperous and free from disturbances.* [30]

> *Anyone who is not lazy in the pursuit of yoga, whether young, old, very old, ill, or weak, attains success through practice.* [31]

Chapter two describes various pranayama, *satkarmas* (cleansing practices, also known as *kriyas*), *kumbhaka* (breath retention), *bandhas* (energetic locks), as well as how to break through the *granthis* (energetic knots).

> *When the breath is disturbed, the mind is unsteady. When the breath becomes focused, the mind becomes focused, and the yogi attains steadiness. Therefore, the breath should be restrained.* [32]

Just like a lion, elephant, or tiger is tamed gradually, the breath too should be brought under control [slowly]. Else it will kill the practitioner.[33]

The mind is the lord of the senses, but the breath is the lord of the mind.[34]

Chapter three discusses *kundalini*, the dormant and very powerful prana at the base of the spine, and *mudras* (gestures or energetic seals) and their benefits.

Just as the Lord of the Serpents (Ananta), is the support of the earth with its mountains and forests, so is kundalini the support of all yoga practices. When the sleeping kundalini awakens, and rises through the grace of the Guru, then all the lotuses and knots (granthis) are pierced.[35]

Chapter four deals with meditation and *samadhi*, spiritual enlightenment, as a journey of personal spiritual growth.

Just as salt dissolves in water, the merging of mind and Self (Atman) is called samadhi. When the prana is restrained and the mind is absorbed [in the Self], that state of harmony is called samadhi.[36]

Place the Self (Atman) in the middle of space (akasa) and space in the midst of the self. Reducing everything to the nature of space, think of nothing else.

Void within, void without, void like a pot in space. Full outside, full like a pot in the ocean. [Such is the state of the yogi in this meditation.]

There should be no thought about external things or any thought about internal things. Relinquishing all such thoughts, [the yogi] should think of nothing.

The entire world is the fabrication of thoughts only. The function of the mind is also created only by thoughts. Transcending the mind, find rest in the changeless. O Rama, then you can attain peace.

Like camphor in fire and like salt in water, the mind dissolves in the true state through meditation (samadhi).[37]

Yoga Sutras of Patanjali

I wanted to focus this part of the book on studying yoga beyond the eight limbs, but that also means understanding the fullness of Patajnali's vision. It's important to note that the Yoga Sutras of Patanjali are a consolidated account of many of the ancient teachings that came before them, including those that were passed down as part of a much older oral tradition. There is much confusion about when they were written, which could be anywhere from 1700 to 2500 years ago.[38]

It's helpful to understand the context of the eight limbs, which Patanjali shares in the middle of the second chapter, the section on how to practice yoga. Before introducing them, he explains that in order to avoid future suffering we need to cultivate discriminative discernment, *viveka khyati.* He goes on to explain that this is achieved by practicing the eight limbs of yoga:

By the practice of the limbs of yoga, the impurities dwindle away and there dawns the light of wisdom, leading to discriminative discernment, viveka khyati.[39]

The eight limbs of yoga are:

1. *Yama*—ethical practices, things not to do
2. *Niyama*—ethical practices, things to do
3. *Asana*—posture or seat
4. *Pranayama*—expansion of *prana*, energy
5. *Pratyahara*—sense withdrawal
6. *Dharana*—concentration
7. *Dhyana*—meditation
8. *Samadhi*—enlightenment

The basic philosophy of the Yoga Sutras of Patanjali is a reflection of earlier teachings found in the Upanishads, but Patanjali uses a more analytical approach. He brilliantly provides a variety of ways to address our "spiritual ignorance," as he would call it. It's almost like he's saying, "Try this technique, and if that doesn't work, try this other one." He also compiles his teachings into lists, which is actually a very modern approach that we still see in contemporary teaching. Look at current articles on yoga, and you'll see endless lists such as, "5 Poses to Reduce Back Pain," or "3 Ways to Reduce Stress."

In particular, Patanjali is sensitive to our suffering, and explains that future pain can be avoided if we cease to identify with our thoughts and connect more deeply with our spirit or true Self. He describes the many obstacles to enlightenment, samadhi, as well as techniques for handling the challenges that humans face due to egoism and selfishness.

In some ways, the Sutras are a manual for the human mind and a guide to experience samadhi. Historians believe that the Yoga Sutras were written for monks who dedicated their lives to the spiritual path. As such, Patanjali is instructing practitioners in leaving the world behind and dedicating themselves to spiritual practice. But for those of us who are firmly planted in this world as householders, there is also much inspiration and guidance that can be gleaned.

Personally, I have been so influenced by the Sutras that I can't talk about yoga without constantly referencing them. In fact, because you'll find so many references to the Sutras throughout this book I'll refrain from quoting more here, although that is challenging for me to do! Instead, I urge you to find a translation that you like, or a few different translations, and consider reading a few sutras regularly as a part of your yoga practice.

Integrating Yoga Philosophy into Class

An essential way to make yoga accessible is to make the subtle, esoteric teachings available and relevant to your students. Of course, this depends on your ability to translate these teachings into practical tools for daily life. It's a challenge for yoga teachers to understand the concepts of yoga clearly enough to be able to share them in meaningful ways, but it's a worthwhile challenge.

Even though the yoga teachings are thousands of years old, they include universal concepts that still provide direction and support for the modern practitioner. The sacred texts describe techniques for working with your mind and finding peace in your life. Your yoga practice can thus allow you to respond to the world in a way that gives you more agency and control. Yoga can provide a means for you to reclaim the peace that the world seems to have taken away.

To share this with your students and bring yoga philosophy into asana-based classes, consider the following possibilities:

- Share a reading directly from the Yoga Sutras, Bhagavad Gita, or other text, and discuss it briefly before class.
- Share an uplifting reading or poem that feels connected to the teachings.
- Integrate a concept from yoga philosophy into class by incorporating ways to practice with that concept in mind. For example,

remind students that ahimsa includes non-violence toward themselves, and ask them to consider their approach to asana with this in mind.

- Give students a homework assignment to practice one of these teachings in their lives. For example, you could ask them to reflect on karma yoga, and to consider how to balance caring for themselves and caring for others.
- Start a book club that focuses on spiritual books and scripture—schedule the book club before or after your yoga class.
- Embody the teachings of yoga in your own life. In fact, by teaching in an accessible and equitable way, you are already embodying yoga ethics and becoming a living example

Scenario

After one of your classes a student comes up to you and says, "I've never met anyone like you. I love your classes so much. I want to learn as much as I can from you. Can you teach me private lessons too?"

Response

There's nothing wrong with someone liking your classes and wanting private lessons. Just be careful. This could be a red flag, or it could just be a person who is very emotive. Strong boundaries are required moving forward. I would respond by asking what they would like to learn in private lessons that we're not covering in group classes, and I would consider offering them private sessions if they seem like they're sincere in their practice.

Further Reflection

- Will you commit to an ongoing study of yoga philosophy?

- Spend time with each of the four texts that I described here. You don't need to study all of them at once. Remember, this is a lifelong journey.

- Consider creating a daily routine of studying just for 10 minutes as part of your regular *sadhana* or daily practice.

- Can you try to apply the teachings in your life?

- Can you begin to make the connection between yoga's ancient philosophical teachings and real-world challenges?

TEACHING AS A PRACTICE

I like the framing of teaching as a practice, because I'm also a student, even if I'm positioned as the teacher. It suggests we're on a path. There's a process, and a journey, and a pathway for this. It's not like I've learned everything I need to learn about whatever topic I'm focused on. We've been conditioned to believe we know more than the people we're teaching. That's how I've been conditioned to think about it. Yet, that's not how I teach because I think that's a flawed model. It sets up a power dynamic that can actually make it difficult for people to learn.

People who have been with me in person will tell you I say, "I don't know," when I truly don't know the answer to a question. I don't make up an answer. I say, "I can ask someone," or "I'm going to go look that up and then come back to the group." I do that all the time.

Humility is such an important way of being in practice for me. How could I know everything, even if I'm positioned as the expert? What I say is that, "I'm learning alongside you all, which means I'm going to make mistakes. I'm not going to know everything." Also, acknowledging that I will make mistakes feels connected to humility and, in my experience, to being a good teacher. That's not often modeled for people. What's typically modeled is to make it up. Make up an answer, pretend you know. Move through it, and past it. Don't actually talk about what's happening in the moment.

I'm a curious person, and something that I've been working with more is wonder. Bringing that into space with me when I'm teaching, especially when we aren't sure how to move forward or through a moment. Bringing in wonder and curiosity feels completely connected to yoga and to teaching. It provides more space for learning—the wonder, the awe, the curiosity. The, "Isn't that interesting?" Not as a way to evade what needs attention, but more as a practice. That feels counter to dominant culture too, to be curious and wonder, "Oh, I've never seen that before."

—Michelle Cassandra Johnson

WHEN I SPOKE with Michelle Cassandra Johnson about teaching as a practice, she reinforced much of what I was thinking. We spoke at length about how the attitude of a teacher informs the experience of the student, and whether a class feels accessible, safe, and welcoming.

In particular, she was clear that humility was the most important characteristic of a yoga teacher. I thought that was compelling considering that if you ask most people, they would probably tell you that the most important characteristic of a yoga teacher is flexibility! In many ways, that's so far from the truth.

If you're not approaching teaching yoga as an ongoing practice, you're approaching it as something that you have already perfected. You make yourself the expert—the one who knows everything. That's a dangerous mountain to climb because there's only one way to go from there, and that's down.

In many ways, humility summarizes all the yoga teachings in one simple concept. Humility means that you are consciously working with your ego-mind, which is what Patanjali has been asking us to do all along. Humility is not self-criticism or self-hatred. Instead, it's a state of mind that is still open to learning and growing. It's a mind that hasn't become so full of itself that there isn't room for anyone else's perspective or ideas to enter.

Reflection

What tone of voice are you using when you talk to yourself, and how might that impact the way you speak to your students?

Self-Awareness as a Practice

The safety and efficacy of your yoga classes depend not only on your knowledge and teaching skills, but also on your sensitivity to your students' experiences both on and off the mat. This includes considering the ways that race, age, disability, sexuality, gender, and other related issues impact every aspect of someone's life. No matter how sensitive you are, your unconscious biases may still make it hard for you to understand how other people may perceive a situation. In the context of a yoga class this means recognizing that you don't always know how an instruction will land.

As a yoga teacher you're working with a diversity of students with a variety of bodies and backgrounds. For example, if you have a student in a group class who has paralysis, how do you give instructions that make them feel included? Do you say, "Lift your right arm… if you can lift your arm." Or is that just insensitive?

The answers to these questions aren't simple. You can work on cultural sensitivity, and reflect on the language you use when teaching, but that's still not enough. The answer to how to make all your students feel welcome and safe is subtler. In the end, it's a question of whether or not you're doing your own practice, and if you're able to see your teaching as an extension of that practice?

It takes a good amount of self-awareness and inner work to be able to recognize that your perspective is just that—only one way of seeing things. While it may not be possible to truly understand someone else's experience, you can at least have enough self-knowledge to admit that your experience is limited. It's not about denying your own truth. Rather, it's allowing your practice to expand your awareness to create space for other peoples' perspectives. So, the answer is that you try your best, and if it doesn't work you learn from your mistakes.

Regarding the student with paralysis, I think the way to approach the situation is with curiosity and care. I would approach the student before class and talk with them about it. What will make that student feel seen and included is completely personal. Generalizations are worthless. One person may want specific instructions for their body, and another may want to fit in and be ignored. In my experience, the best approach is to simply ask, "How can I support you in this class today?"

Reflection

Do you perceive teaching as an ongoing practice or do you feel that you have to have all the answers?

Ease as a Practice

I recently saw a reel on Instagram with a young yoga teacher performing almost impossibly challenging asanas. In a voiceover, he proclaimed that we should, "Make yoga hard," and he went on to say that we should, "Find a strict teacher who will show us the power of discipline and keep us in line."

I understand the importance of discipline and *tapas*, which is learning from our challenges and struggles. But, as humans, most of us have enough challenges in our lives already—especially marginalized folks. In fact, most people come to yoga to find a way out of pain.

The ascetic approach to yoga, which is a thread in yoga history, has been embraced by capitalism and modern society as an individualistic way to attain some kind of personal liberation, but it's a lie. Our liberation is tied together. As Fannie Lou Hamer, the civil rights activist, famously said, "Nobody's free until everybody's free."

Plus, is that the kind of teacher you want to be? A strict teacher who keeps your students in line? We've already seen that approach in many traditional yoga lineages where the guru used intimidation and abuse; it has no place in our contemporary practice. Your students won't find freedom from being encouraged to punish themselves or shame themselves into submission, and you won't find peace in being the all-powerful disciplinarian.

Your students will find freedom from loving themselves completely and fully just as they are. In fact, loving the parts of themselves that they're most ashamed of is the true path to wholeness and healing. There's nothing wrong with a structured or disciplined practice, but if students are pushing themselves out of some unconscious desire for your approval, or because you're shaming them, then that's not yoga, it's abuse.

Avoiding Being Judgmental as a Practice

Sometimes we push or shame our students because of our own insecurities as a teacher. So, it's important to practice not being judgmental. The next time you meet a new student try to watch how your mind jumps to conclusions about them. Instead, see if you can pause and question the judgments you make about them. Notice how it feels to simply exist with another being knowing that their heart and your heart are the same even though they beat inside very different bodies with completely different minds.

Time and time again, I see the ways my mind makes up stories and judgments about people. I can think of so many students who surprised me over the years. I remember one student who always seemed disappointed by me and by our time together. She would rush out at the end of class, and always had a look of concern on her face. I kept thinking she would stop coming to class, but she didn't. Over time, I started to realize that I was projecting this disappointment onto her. Students with larger bodies, older students, disabled students, and students of color often express their frustration about yoga teachers assuming that they are inexperienced when they attend class.

Surprisingly, I noticed my tendency to judge my students seemed to get worse the more experienced I became. After teaching for a while, I started to intuit things about my students. I could see how someone moved their body and get a feeling for the way it reflected what was happening with them mentally or emotionally. But that still didn't mean I understood their experience. It was just my feeling.

Patanjali even talks about this as a *siddhi*, or power, that can be achieved by practice. In book three of his Yoga Sutras, he describes some of the benefits that come with intensive practice. He explains:

> *By samyama (intensive meditation) on the distinguishing signs of others' bodies, knowledge of their mental images is obtained. But this does not include the support in the person's mind [such as the motive behind the thought, etc.] as that is not the object of the samyama.*[40]

In other words, if you're a very experienced teacher you may get intuitive hits about what's happening with your students physically. But, you can't know what is going on inside their hearts or minds. It is an easy trap to fall into. Getting an intuitive feeling about what's going on with a student is a gift, and can inspire your teaching. But you have to be thoughtful about how you present that information.

Sometimes, I notice something about a student, usually it's in the form of a feeling. I might feel slightly anxious or sad around them. Rather than make an assumption that the feeling is coming from them, I simply ask them how they're feeling, or use it as a prompt for the group. I might ask the group if they can use today's practice to process feelings and move energy.

Avoiding Spiritual Bypassing as a Practice

One of the challenges of being a yoga teacher is that people seem to think we are perfect, enlightened beings. On the contrary, I find yoga teachers are often people who are really struggling with life, but are doing it in a conscious way. Believing the lie—that yoga teachers have to be "above it all," or allow "good vibes only"—is spiritual bypassing, which is the use of spiritual teachings to avoid painful or negative emotions.

It can also happen in a subtler way when I avoid my negative or painful emotions in the name of spirituality. Or, when I use spiritual concepts like oneness or karma to avoid seeing the suffering of others. The fact is, yoga is not an escape from reality, but a deep dive into it.

For me, avoiding spiritual bypassing means facing reality head on and accepting that pain and suffering are part of life. By doing so, by embracing my own suffering, I find compassion for your suffering. But the reality is that it's the hardest part of my practice—although it may be the most important. If I don't do it, I'm basically living in a fantasy of denial.

At least in my experience, a healthy, integrated spiritual life begins by acknowledging pain and letting painful emotions exist and move through me. Then, I can work on finding more love and compassion for myself and for you. That's the beauty of having a yoga practice after all.

Spiritual bypassing can also be an obstacle to yoga. Of course, tons of people mistakenly think, "I'm not flexible enough to do yoga." But there are many others who may feel like they're just too mentally or emotionally unstable to do yoga. They probably don't see themselves reflected in the serene marketing imagery of the yoga industry that often depicts someone calmly sitting in full lotus on a mountain top or blissfully doing a fancy pose on a beach.

This may be especially true for those who have mental health challenges. This is a particularly unfortunate misconception, since the practice can be so beneficial for mental health if it's approached honestly and with realistic expectations. We have this strange idea that if you practice or teach yoga you have to live a pure, "natural," lifestyle, and this false idea may keep people from the practice. I've even heard yoga teachers shame people for taking prescription medications for their mental health. The idea that yoga practitioners don't take medications is a subtle and powerful form of spiritual bypassing and ableism.

Most people come to yoga because they are in some kind of pain, whether it's psychological, physical, or even spiritual. And while yoga can offer tremendous healing and transformation, that healing doesn't occur through denial of the reality of our lives or the reality of our suffering. On the contrary, it is through radical honesty and acceptance that healing happens.

Reflection

How do I integrate the spiritual teachings of yoga with my lived human experience?

Imperfectionism as a Practice

When I'm training yoga teachers, I often hear them talk about feeling overwhelmed by the amount of knowledge they think they must have in order to make yoga accessible to all their students. They also worry about being able to provide variations of practices to each individual student within a group class. This is both wonderful and concerning. The urge to make their offerings accessible is wonderful, but the sense of overwhelm can be paralyzing, and feed into a kind of perfectionism.

I think this perfectionism can originate from wanting to truly serve others and be the best teacher possible. It also connects to the desire to not cause harm, which is the foundational teaching of yoga. But there is another side to it. That is the ego not wanting to be wrong or make a mistake. It's the hallmark of our human fragility and fear. The worry is that I'll look stupid or embarrass myself. Of course, I've made many mistakes and embarrassed myself many times—and I've survived! In fact, I've learned more from those public mistakes than from any other training or experience I could have had.

The other essential element to letting go of perfectionism and control is to practice humility, and reflect on the fact that you are really just a vehicle for teachings that have literally existed for millenia. This doesn't mean that you aren't responsible for what you do and what you say, but it is a good reminder that you didn't create yoga, and you are simply sharing what you've learned.

ABCs of Accessible Yoga

One essential point to remember is that 100 percent accessibility isn't possible to achieve, and there are many reasons for this. One reason is that we can't always tell from outside what support or accommodations a student may need, and they may not always tell you. Teaching

Accessible Yoga isn't about figuring out how to teach twenty different versions of a practice for your twenty students. Rather, it's about learning skills and techniques that allow all twenty students to find their own practice in the midst of the group class. That is an important distinction.

There are specific skills that yoga teachers can learn to make their offerings accessible to everyone. In fact, these techniques are typically more effective at achieving accessibility than individually teaching each student would be. That's because these skills are about giving students agency and choice. They're about educating them to connect with what they are experiencing and begin to figure out what they need themselves. The process of teaching, providing real education, is more about this long-term path than the short term solution of simply telling everyone what to do.

Another reason why 100 percent accessibility isn't achievable is because students within a class may have opposing needs. One may want the room colder and one may want it warmer. These needs may be based not just on personal desire but on their health or disability. It's not possible to create a perfect environment where no one ever gets disturbed or upset. We do our best, but some friction is unavoidable. In this situation, you may need to work together as a team and collaborate to find a solution. So often the key to accessibility lies not in the endless knowledge of a teacher, but in their skill at sharing power.

To make practices accessible, keep the ABCs of Accessible Yoga in mind: Agency, Boundaries, and Collaboration.

> **Agency**—Make sure students know they can opt out or adapt as they like.

> **Boundaries**—Students need to respect each other's boundaries, so while they are each encouraged to find their own practice, it can't harm or interfere with another student's experience.

Collaboration—If there are conflicting needs in a space, you can bring students together to collaborate and find a solution.

Community as a Practice

Often when I teach about how collaboration supports accessibility, I'm usually referring to a collaboration between teacher and student, which can be incredibly powerful. But there is also the collaboration that happens within a group of students. They can support and encourage each other in essential ways. So it's important to reflect on how you can help to build a positive yoga community that is supportive, welcoming, and safe for all your students.

When I spoke to Michelle Cassandra Johnson, she explained how community building is an outcome of humility because it shifts power from the individual teacher to the group. It's an acknowledgment of the healing power of the community. I love the idea that a yoga community is more than its lead teacher or teachers. It is the community itself that is key. It reminds me of Thich Nhat Hanh's famous saying, "The next Buddha will be a sangha."[41]

Personally, I find group classes to be a very different experience from my home practice. The group offers support and encouragement and a sense of comradery that inspires and motivates me. Cultivating a healthy community is one of the truly special opportunities of teaching yoga.

The stereotype of a lone yogi sitting in meditation in a cave is more mythology than reality. Community is itself a yoga practice because it's about learning to see yourself in others—which can be hard to do. This idea of transcending our individualism is a thread woven throughout the history of yoga. You can even see it in the wisdom of the *Bhagavad Gita*:

As your mind becomes harmonized through yoga practices, you begin to see the Atman in all beings and all beings in your Self; you see the same Self everywhere and in everything.[42]

Ironically, to facilitate the inward journey of the yoga path, we need outer support. Support in the form of a loving community. Sangha, spiritual community, is helpful in inspiring practice as well as keeping us on the path when we're struggling. This can be a lot simpler than it sounds. It can simply be a group of students who become yoga friends, bound together by a welcoming teacher.

While we all benefit from community, Accessible Yoga classes may include students who are particularly isolated. Isolation can be unhealthy mentally and physically, so creating opportunities for community-building is not only a nice idea, but a very effective technique for supporting students in general. As a teacher, consider ways to support connection and community. This could include:

- Having students introduce themselves at the beginning of class or doing a quick icebreaker.
- Learning your regular students' names.
- Creating space before or after class for conversation.
- Encouraging students to support each other. They can connect and form friendships outside of class in a way that may not be appropriate for you as the teacher.
- Thinking of activities for the students to do together, such as form a book group, or create a fundraiser for a cause they are interested in supporting.

Scenario

You have a new student who is older and has some mobility challenges. They approach you after class and say, "I would really like more of a work out. Can you push us a little harder?"

Response

Interestingly, this has happened to me numerous times. My classes tend to be very gentle, and I focus on the subtle aspects of yoga. I realize this isn't for everyone. But I also realize that many people aren't ready for slow and subtle. So I see two ways to address this.

1. Help this student understand what yoga is really about. Use this as a teaching opportunity to show them that slowing down and being more mindful is actually a key element of yoga practice. I sometimes do this during class by turning the students' competitive nature back on itself. I might say something like, "Let's see who can move slowest coming out of this pose." This is also an opportunity to ask the student what their goals are in practicing yoga. They may not realize that there are tremendous health benefits to slowing down and connecting with themselves.
2. Take the feedback for what it is without getting defensive. That could mean giving the student more challenging variations of the practices you're already doing, recommending they hold the poses longer, or simply helping them find a different

teacher who teaches a more intensive physical practice.

Further Reflection

- Can you commit to being a lifelong student of yoga?

- Are you willing to keep your ego in check by finding peer support, or other methods such as regular therapy, to help keep you grounded?

- Do you approach challenges as an opportunity for deeper learning?

- Are you patient with yourself? Do you allow yourself to be a beginner?

TEACHING ASANA

CHAPTER FIVE

POWER & CONSENT

In any relationship there's a power dynamic, and that's no different in yoga spaces. As teachers, we hold disproportionate power in the student-teacher dynamic, and wherever we hold disproportionate power, I think we also own disproportionate responsibility that comes along with that. So, I think we're responsible for recognizing the power dynamics at play in yoga class, and also for mitigating the ways in which they can disempower our students.

I don't think we do that by needlessly giving away our own power, though. I don't think we can just abdicate the responsibilities, or their accompanying privileges, that come with the role of teacher. I can't just give up the role of teacher. I also can't just give up my white privilege. It's going to exist because of dominant culture and the way society enforces that. But instead of giving away our own power, I think we can leverage our power and use it to create more access for our students, particularly access to their own innate power and resources.

I think this means using our power to make more resources available in the room, which could be options for practice or variations of postures. It could be props. I also think it involves a sharing of voice, ensuring that our students have an equitable share of voice in the room and that their needs and desires are heard, respected, and hopefully met. I think we also need to *look at the ways we're privileged within dominant culture, and work to leverage that power toward equity and accessibility in the room, rather than intentionally or unintentionally wielding it over students with oppressed and marginalized identities that we don't hold.*

—M Camellia

FOR MANY REASONS, being a yoga teacher can feel confusing. On the one hand, you have knowledge of the practices and experience practicing and teaching. The student probably has less experience and knowledge of yoga, but they do have knowledge of themselves. The student has their own inner wisdom and knowing. So the paradox is that you have knowledge and they have wisdom. That's potentially the perfect combination to create the alchemy of yoga, but it can be a delicate balance. In the end, our job isn't so much to teach yoga but to guide the student to become their own teacher.

In the Bhagavad Gita, Krishna talks about the difference between a wise and unwise person, which feels important for yoga teachers to consider. He explains that an unwise or unenlightened person simply has more attachments than the wise person. Attachment, *vairagya*, refers to our relationship to the things in the world that we mistakenly think we need to be happy. As teachers, our job isn't just doing longer meditations or more complicated asanas. Our job is to release our attachments and to guide students by example. He explains:

The unenlightened do things with attachment (wanting some results for themselves). An enlightened person does things with the same zeal, Arjuna, but without attachment, and thus guides others on the path of selfless action (karma yoga). A wise person will not disturb the mind of an unwise person who is still attached to the fruits of their actions. But by continuously performing perfect (selfless) actions the wise person influences others in all they do.[45]

When a new student comes to you, do you see problems that need to be fixed: A "bad" back, a hunched spine, a stressed mind? Is your goal to change them, improve them, make them "better?" What kind of relationship starts like that—with only seeing the other person's limitations? No matter how skilled you are as a yoga teacher or yoga therapist, you're not going to heal anyone from anything. They might heal themselves with your guidance, but that's on them, not you.

A student once shared a story about his experience with another yoga teacher. He uses a wheelchair, and hesitantly went to a yoga class. The teacher immediately pounced on him and, rather than asking him questions, started to make claims about the benefits of yoga. She even had the nerve to tell him that if he attended her classes regularly she would help him walk again!

This was wrong on so many levels. The most insidious thing about that teacher's statement was that she assumed that the student wanted to walk. She had no idea why he was using a wheelchair or what using the wheelchair meant to him. Let's just say that he almost gave up on yoga after that experience.

This story reminds me of the ways we use language. For example, saying someone is "wheelchair bound" or "bed bound" makes an assumption about their relationship to the supports they're using. Most wheelchair users that I know say that they consider their chair a source of freedom, not limitation.

If your goal is to fix your students, you'll be fighting an uphill battle. Life brings illness, disability, and eventually death. It's unavoidable. While yoga provides tremendous benefits, it's dangerous to bring a strictly therapeutic approach to a spiritual practice. It can create confusion and often is based on ableism and healthism. While it's natural to want to reduce your students' suffering, it's important to reflect on where that desire comes from.

Reflection

Do you assume your older students are trying to regain their youth, larger-bodied students are trying to lose weight, or disabled students want to be fixed or healed?

Agency

If you see your students as already whole and full, you are cultivating a very different relationship with them than you would be if your intention were to fix or change them. Plus, if you start taking responsibility for your students' healing, how will you feel when they get sick or die? Think of the burden you are carrying, and how much pressure you are putting on yourself. I found that taking on that responsibility was burning me out.

Early in my teaching journey many of my students with AIDS passed away. Each loss was devastating and made me question what I was doing, but somehow I found the will to keep teaching. Then just a few years ago, I was working with a young woman who had an unusually severe form of multiple sclerosis. Each week when she would come to class, she would have worsened symptoms, and she was really struggling. I felt completely powerless, and wasn't sure how to help her.

So, I approached one of my yoga teacher friends to ask him what else I could do to support her. He stopped me, and simply said, "You're making it about you." It was such a great example of how helpful peer support is. His reflection made me see the situation in a different way. This student's journey was hers, and I was judging it and deciding how it should go. Once I was able to let go of my desire to control, I realized that her journey of illness and wellness was hers only. I was just supporting her personal evolution. Soon afterwards she passed away and it was very upsetting, but my friend's insight made it more bearable for me.

Building your students' agency means encouraging them to each listen to their own inner voice, their intuition, and their inner wisdom. That's the way they can access the true power of yoga. I often tell my students, "Listen to me, but don't listen to me." Hear the words that I'm saying, but follow your inner guidance.

The other day, during class, a student asked me, "How should this feel?" That question is the sign of an open mind, which I appreciate. But it also speaks to their desire to do it "right," to fit in, and potentially, to their expectation that growth will happen in a particular way. I responded to the student with, "You tell me. What are you feeling?"

Interoception, which I'll discuss in detail on page 130, is the sense of what is happening inside the body, and can be cultivated through yoga practice. By bringing their awareness within, students can create more capacity to listen to that inner voice, respond to those inner sensations, and practice in a way that is in alignment with what they're feeling in the moment. That's the mark of an experienced practitioner—increased sensitivity to their inner world, not increased sensitivity to a teacher's instructions.

Some ways to encourage that inner journey in your students is to invite them to listen to themselves, to identify the sensations that they're experiencing as they practice, to do body scans, and bring awareness to different parts of the body in a neutral, non-judgmental way. That last point alone is transformational. Asking them to notice how they feel before and after they do a particular practice can be very effective in increasing self-awareness. Also, helping students become aware of the way they talk to themselves can be a lifelong gift.

Reflection

Is it difficult for you to sit with your students' suffering? Do you feel like a failure if they come to your classes and don't have less suffering?

Consent

As a teacher, it's your responsibility to engage in and model good consent practices. Consent, briefly defined, is, "permission for something to happen." That "something" may certainly be touch (such as for the use of hands-on assists). But consent also applies beyond physical contact.

For example, registering for and showing up to class is often regarded as consent to participate in the yoga you're offering. This means that practicing informed consent with your students begins even before they enter your class. You can do this by ensuring the accuracy of your class description, bio, and other marketing materials. Clear class descriptions are essential for accessibility so students know what the class entails. They are also trauma-sensitive, because they allow students to be aware of what to expect in your class.

According to yoga teacher, M Camellia, who I interviewed for this chapter, in order to have consent, all four of these elements must be present:

1. Clear: There must be a shared language and open communication between you and your student in order for consent to be given. This may be verbal, written, or signified via nonverbal cues (such as a head nod or thumbs up) as long as the meaning of those cues is clearly understood by both teacher and student. This also applies when you use a translator for

students who speak a different language and for students who use assistive devices to speak.

2. Coherent: If your student loses consciousness, falls asleep, or is otherwise incapacitated, they cannot give consent.

3. Willing: Even if someone indicates agreement, that agreement is not actually consent if it is forced, coerced, given under false pretenses, or given under the pressure of a power imbalance. Willingness requires both specific, accurate information about what your intended action is (e.g., "May I place my hand between your shoulder blades to bring awareness to your spine?"), and the ability to freely say "yes" or "no" without fear of judgment or retribution.

4. Ongoing: Consent must be obtained for every step of an interaction and can be revoked at any time, for any reason. Even if your student said "yes" to an assist earlier, you still need to request informed consent again before assisting them again. If you are in the middle of an assist and the student asks you to stop, stop immediately and check in.[44]

It's important to note that consent cannot be given by a caretaker or aide on behalf of a student, although that caretaker may be able to assist with communication. It's also important to acknowledge that there is an inherent power dynamic at play between student and teacher. As the person in the position of power within your classes, it's your responsibility to ensure you hold yourself accountable and practice sharing power with your students, allowing them agency over their bodies, their practice, and their time and space.

You can share power with your students by offering invitations instead of commands, intentionally providing options and opportunities for choice-making, and by fostering an ongoing awareness of your social positioning and the ways your social privileges (white privilege, thin privilege, privilege based on physical ability, etc.) may have an impact on the power dynamics in your classes.

Language & Power

According to British writer Angela Carter, "Language is power, life and the instrument of culture, the instrument of domination and liberation."[45] As yoga teachers, our goal may be liberation for our students, but are we speaking to them with language that dominates or liberates?

Since language is the main vehicle for our teaching, we need to be conscious of the words we choose, and how we use them. Throughout this book, I explore different aspects of the power dynamics that exist between teacher and student and how an awareness of these dynamics is an essential ingredient in making yoga accessible. So, let's take a moment to reflect on our language choices in general.

A friend of mine is an advanced Iyengar Yoga instructor, and I once asked her why teachers in her tradition seem to have a similar, rather assertive, way of giving verbal instructions in their classes. She told me that they are trained to, "Speak directly to the body and bypass the mind." I was struck by that comment, because on the one hand it makes sense. Much of yoga practice is about bypassing the mind and working directly with the body or the breath. Through practice, the body's experience is amplified so that the thoughts fade into the background.

But is that an experience that can be cultivated by the teacher through their tone of voice, and more specifically through the use of commanding language? Personally, I had the opposite experience in Iyengar classes. I appreciated the clear instruction, but I found it to be overly restrictive and controlling. Of course my experience is just that, and everyone has different reactions to the way they are spoken to.

Personally, I feel like I want to be spoken to in a polite, gentle, and clear way. So I try to speak to my students that way. There is a delicate balance between gentleness and clarity that I am always seeking. If I'm too vague it often leads to confused looks. I believe that teaching in a way that invites students to find their own practice is essential, yet they also need safety and clear direction, especially if they are relatively new to the practice.

This question comes up for me when I hear some trauma-sensitive teachers advocate for always using invitational language. Generally speaking, invitational language is great, but for new students, asking them to constantly explore how they feel can be downright confusing and ineffective. Personally, I like to give general instructions about finding your own practice in the beginning of a class, and remind students of that a few times throughout the class. Then within each practice I offer at least two clear options to choose from and make my instructions as concise as possible.

Politeness and gentleness are also completely subjective. I've been to classes where every single instruction was given with a "Please," and it started to get irritating. If I come to your class, I want you to teach me. You can remind me that it's my practice, and that yoga is about increased sensitivity to my internal experience—but not in every sentence! What's even more important for me is a feeling of connection, shared humanity, and respect, all of which can be cultivated through language.

One of the most important things to keep in mind regarding language is that most students are literally hanging on your every word. If you spend a lot of time introducing a practice or give a ton of detailed instructions, it can be hard for them to know what to do. I've been in classes where the teacher spent five minutes introducing a pose and during that time I wasn't sure if I was supposed to be practicing the pose or just sitting and listening to them lecture. In addition to keeping your instructions clear and concise in general, it's also essential to communicate exactly when the students come into and out of a practice.

Sometimes, as teachers, we get lost in the details in our heads, or we feel like we're on stage giving a performance. Focusing on serving the students in front of you is the most important way to share power. Our verbal instructions need to be based on keen observation.

Observation is an essential tool that will help you create a safe and welcoming environment.

For example, if you're teaching a flow, such as sun salutation, and you notice one student is confused or lagging behind, what do you do? Do you just keep going hoping that they will eventually figure it out, or do you slow down and adapt your instruction to allow them to catch up? Also, if you see someone doing something incorrectly or in a potentially dangerous way, how do you call them out? Do you say their name or point them out and tell them they're wrong, or do you repeat the instruction to the entire class and make a general correction so they don't feel shamed?

Reflection

Are you offering instruction in a way that is simultaneously respectful and clear? How could you potentially improve upon this?

Inclusive Language

Awareness of our language, cuing, and word choice is essential when teaching, and can help students feel welcome and seen. For example, someone who can't raise their arms overhead might appreciate instructions that are inclusive such as "raise your arms up as far as comfortable" instead of "raise your arms up alongside your head" which they may not be able to do.

Of course, we all make mistakes, and the point is to do your best without obsessing over every word that comes out of your mouth. Sometimes we overcompensate and infantilize our students, especially older adults, by speaking in overly concerned or worried tones. An example of this is using the word "just" as in "just raise your arms up in front of you," even though you may be saying it to sound sensitive. It can come across as belittling.

Notice if you tend to give a lot of warnings and raise concerns in your instructions. There are contraindications for every practice, but you could spend an entire class talking about them and the student may come away more worried than when they arrived. If possible, find a way to provide some essential contraindications in a way that doesn't raise alarm or stress. For example, "If you're not practicing a full inversion because of high blood pressure or glaucoma, you're welcome to invert part of the body in legs up the wall, or legs on a chair pose."

The nocebo effect is the opposite of the placebo effect—which is the positive effect attributed to our belief about something. The nocebo effect occurs when negative expectations are set. For example, if I was teaching an inversion and I said, "This practice might make you dizzy," and all of a sudden my suggestion makes you feel dizzy. So you need to find a way to share essential contraindications or warnings without putting negative thoughts into people's minds. Of course, satya, truthfulness, is the key to this.

Using Sanskrit

In order to lessen cultural appropriation, it's important to make an effort to include and respect traditional practices such as chanting or reading from yoga philosophy texts. This is a way to respect and to share the deeper teachings of yoga with your students. But not everyone is open to this and some students may have a strong reaction.

In terms of accessibility, it's important that if you use Sanskrit in your classes—which also includes using the Sanskrit names of poses —you always translate the Sanskrit as well. Just using Sanskrit names of poses without translation, or leading a chant without explaining what it means, does often feel exclusive and potentially unwelcoming. To me, this is just another aspect of my job as a yoga educator.

Teaching people Sanskrit words is a great way to share more about yoga history and culture. You could say, "Next we'll practice tree pose, *vrksasana*." Or, "This traditional mantra means, 'May all beings be at peace. *Lokah samastah sukhino bhavantu.*'"

There is another aspect to the question of Sanskrit usage that is even more complicated. In the caste system of India, access to Sanskrit, both spoken or written, was limited to higher castes. That meant that lower caste people were not allowed to hear, speak, or read Sanskrit, and could be tortured or killed if they did.

In an interview where she was asked about her experience with Sanskrit in yoga classes, Dalit rights activist Thenmozhi Soundararajan described being forced to chant in a yoga class. She explained:

> *Sanskrit was weaponized by the Brahmin class… We were not allowed to speak it. We weren't even allowed to listen to it. Otherwise, we'd have our tongues cut off and lead poured in our ears. So it was very troubling to be in a [yoga] class and have a teacher say to me, 'You can't really get the benefits of this practice if you don't do the mantra, and you have to do it,' And if I didn't, then I was going to be asked to leave the class.*[46]

So the question of whether or not to use Sanskrit in a yoga class is extremely complicated. It needs to be approached with thoughtfulness and care. On the one hand, we need to respect tradition and expose our students to the heart of the practice of yoga. At the same time, for many students, using Sanskrit can be inaccessible and even triggering.

Person-First vs. Identity-First Language

We all have the right to choose how we want people to refer to us. In the past, it was considered polite to use person-first language when talking to or about disabled people. An example is "a person with a disability." But, language changes quickly, and over the past few years there has been a major shift toward identity-first language such as a "disabled person," "Deaf person," or an "autistic person."[47] And that is the language I'm using in this book.

It's always best to ask someone the language they prefer, or simply avoid referencing someone's disability until they mention it. Of course there are many people who still prefer person-first language, but one universal agreement I hear from disabled people is that euphemisms for disability are offensive. That includes terms like "differently-abled," or "special needs."

Pronouns

In order to respect the diversity of human experience and identity, it's essential to use the correct pronouns when talking to, or about, someone. In order to make all students more comfortable with sharing pronouns, make it a habit of introducing yourself with your own pronouns (i.e., "Hello, I'm Jivana and my pronouns are he/him/his").

Not everyone is comfortable sharing their pronouns, so forcing the issue is not helpful. If someone doesn't choose to share their pronouns with you it's generally safest to only use their name, or use they/them/theirs which is the most neutral form of pronouns in English.[48] Of course, this question of pronoun usage applies only to languages that use gendered pronouns.

Gendered Language

Stereotypes are harmful and offensive to marginalized communities. They can make people feel invisible and help to keep oppressive systems in place. Yoga classes are places intended to help people relax and turn inward. Therefore, the most neutral language is best.

To build safer spaces, avoid using any kind of gender stereotypes in your teaching, such as "men have tight hamstrings." Gender-related stereotypes like this can make some students feel left out or unseen. Similarly, referring to the class with gendered language, such as "guys" or "ladies" will make the space unwelcoming and exclusive. Instead, you could use phrases such as "everyone," "y'all," "friends," or "people."

Pronouns & Perspective

Another ongoing debate in yoga teaching is whether we should use the possessive "you" and "your" when talking about parts of the body, or if we should use a more neutral "the." For example, is it preferable to say, "Raise your arms overhead," or "Raise the arms overhead?"

While this seems like a minor point, it becomes a major issue in the tone of the entire class. Yoga teachers have strong feelings about this point and go deep into the philosophical meaning of possessive pronouns. Some say that by not using possessive pronouns, it offers students a chance to reflect on whether they identify with the body or the spirit. So perhaps using "the" has a place if we're following traditional aspects of a dualistic yoga philosophy that teach us to disengage from the body, which is part of nature.

But this can also lead to a sense of separation or even dissociation which seems unproductive for most contemporary practitioners. In a way, we need to get back into the body before we can let it go. This is a more trauma-sensitive approach. When I teach I tend to go back and forth between "the" and "your," according to what flows best in that moment, but in general, I find myself leaning toward "your." There is so much healing potential that can happen when we bring our present moment awareness into our bodies rather than distracting ourselves.

Contemporary culture is constantly pulling at our attention. Our phones have become appendages draining our inner battery. Yoga provides an opportunity to recharge in the most profound way. We can connect to a source of infinite energy within us. As much as possible, I want my teaching to draw people closer and closer to that internal power. This occurs when we sense a feeling of connection with our whole selves: Body, mind, and spirit. Separating from the body may not actually be the quickest route to spirit. Rather, integration feels like a healthier and more effective strategy.

It's also useful to reflect on pronoun usage in terms of the efficacy of your instructions. Some teachers use first person "I" statements when teaching. They may say things like, "I'm lifting my arms," with the intention that students should follow along. Some teachers use first person language but in a slightly different way. They may frame it almost as a request, saying something such as, "I'd like you to lift your arms." I also often hear third person "we" statements, such as, "Next, we'll lift our arms."

As I shared above, second person "you" statements are also effective. For example, "Lift your arms." To me that is the simplest and most direct way of teaching, but all of these are viable options. In the end it's really your personal choice. What is important is to reflect on what language you are using and make conscious decisions about it and how it shifts the tone of your teaching.

Scenario

You have a student named Joe who has come to your classes for many years. A newer student named Beth approaches you after class and says that after last week's class Joe asked her out, and she's not interested. Beth says she doesn't feel comfortable coming back to class if Joe is there. What do you say?

Response

This is a very challenging situation, and your response is dependent on the severity of the situation. If Beth feels like she's being harassed by Joe, then you need to ask him to stop coming to class. But, if Joe approached her once and asked her out in a polite, non-threatening way, and he accepted her response, then that has not reached the level of sexual harassment. It still might make Beth feel more comfortable if you spoke with Joe and told him to be sure not to approach Beth again. So it's best to ask Beth what kind of support she needs from you.[49]

Further Reflection

- Reflect on your personal relationship with consent.

- Have you been in relationships where you have crossed another person's boundaries?

- Or have you been on the receiving end of a relationship where the other person crossed your boundaries and/or ignored your needs?

- Reflect on ways that you can ensure that you are receiving your students' consent when you're teaching them.

- Consider how your classes encourage your students' personal agency.

- Consider recording yourself teaching and watching it back so you can hear your word choice and general tone.

- Study more about the history of Sanskrit and decide if you feel comfortable using it.

- Talk to your disabled students about the language they prefer.

CHAPTER SIX

CREATING ACCESSIBLE OFFERINGS

We may want to make our classes available for "all levels," or make our classes accessible for folks who are practicing on a mat or in a chair, but if true accessibility is our aim, there's still more to consider—beyond offering physical accommodations and pose variations. I think about myself as a Trans person. As yoga teachers, we want to include Trans people in our classes and make sure they feel safe and welcomed, etc. But, sometimes our intention doesn't match the impact.

Who are we actually prepared to teach? What is our scope of practice as teachers? We're not going to be for every student. That's okay. But I think we need to be transparent about where we are in our own learning and our own unlearning. I think that when we simply say, "All are welcome," sometimes that's not actually true.

This is the part that can feel mismatched. Sometimes our marketing can signal inclusion and accessibility. But if we're not actually prepared to back up that signaling with creating change and action in the spaces that we're holding, then we're more likely to actually exclude people while intending to be inclusive.

For me, given where I'm at in my personal practice right now, I don't, in general, feel comfortable practicing with cisgender yoga teachers. That's just me personally. So while I understand and believe that cisgender yoga teachers have a responsibility to understand how to make their spaces more welcoming for Trans students, my nervous system will not relax into the practice when I feel that there are unchecked power dynamics. Or when I feel like I can't trust someone to hold the space intentionally, or meaningfully, or with great care.

I think that there is a big misconception in yoga that people have the right to just put their hands on students' bodies without consent. In fact there are many misconceptions which have led to a lack of safety for me in my practice, at least when practicing in public classes. I think that we as teachers should do our due diligence to make ourselves available for all students, all bodies, and all "levels." I also think we need to accept that some students aren't going to connect with us, and that we're not going to be for everybody. Both things are true.

—Tristan Katz

IT'S NOT UNCOMMON to experience a yoga class where the teacher stands at the front of the room barking out orders while the students all follow along in a robotic fashion. Or, a class where the teacher is doing some kind of asana performance at the front of the room, barely paying attention to the students, as if on stage.

The energy in these rooms can be competitive or performance focused. Often the students try their best to look like the other people in the class, not only by following along with the exact same variations of the practice, but by actually physically looking like, or dressing like, the other students. They may be afraid to stand out or be different in any way.

As a student, I've fallen into this trap myself. In fact, the only times I've ever been injured in yoga has been in public classes. In my home practice, I can turn my awareness inward and practice with care. But in a group, I tend to focus on what everyone else is doing—even though I have been practicing for so many years. Since this is something I have had a hard time letting go of, I have a feeling it is true of others as well.

These competitive environments make the teacher's attention a valuable resource. Students are excited to get praised or scared of being criticized or singled out. This can mimic school environments, where the teacher holds all the power. As a teacher, you may fall into this role out of insecurity or because you were literally trained this way. Also, students might believe, incorrectly, that this is how yoga is done. They may think, "My job is to conform and comply. My job is to make pretty shapes with my body to achieve athletic performance and to please the teacher."

We also don't know what kind of past trauma students are bringing to the yoga room. Many of us have been trained by society to conform to the extreme. Some people may feel like their lives literally depend on doing what everyone else is doing, while others are seeking attention and approval.

Reflection

How do you respond to a student who needs a lot of extra attention?

It may be useful to spend some time considering how you respond in group yoga classes. Do you seek to blend in, or do you want attention? Do you worry about what other people are thinking of you? Are you waiting on the teacher to give you some praise?

With more knowledge of your own conditioning, and the ways that you behave within a yoga class, you can begin to reflect on how to make the classes as effective as possible for your students. Remember, that doesn't necessarily mean pleasing them. It means teaching them how to practice yoga in a way that is safe and effective.

Financial Accessibility

Accessibility is multifaceted. It is affirmed through conscious representation of those who have been unwelcome and excluded. It is about overcoming the obstacles to access, including all aspects of white supremacy, such as racism, cultural appropriation, fatphobia, ageism, ableism, and more.

As an individual teacher this may feel overwhelming, but the question is: "What can I do? What steps can I personally take to make yoga more accessible?" It can be helpful to break down all the elements of a yoga class to look at where there may be obstacles to access. For example, is the class financially affordable? Finances are a huge obstacle, and one that is rarely discussed. Online classes, especially free and low cost ones, have helped. But there is still a lot of work to be done in this area.

One way to make your classes more financially accessible is to have tiered pricing and scholarships. Tiered pricing is where you make three or more different price points available for an offering. The middle tier is your regular price, and then you have a lower, discounted rate, and a higher rate for those who want to support those paying the lower rate.

This technique relies on students choosing the tier that is most appropriate for their financial status. I use this for all my offerings and estimate that about 40 percent choose the low and middle option, and about 20 percent choose the higher tier. So, I accept that the average will be slightly lower than the regular price. But, this model usually allows more people to attend.

Providing scholarships is also crucial. These can be either partial, full, or both. The challenge that I found with scholarships is the amount of time it takes to process them. In my trainings, in order to reduce the time to administer them, we automated the process. People answer a series of questions, and based on their responses will get an automatic scholarship offer.

Another challenging thing about scholarships is deciding who to give them to. It can be difficult to choose one person over another. So, it's essential that you work out the requirements for scholarships ahead of time so that you can avoid that situation. Another way to handle this is to decide that you'll have a certain number of scholarships available for your class series, or workshop, or training, and dedicate them to particular communities, such as three scholarships for BIPOC, and three scholarships for LGBTQIA+ or disabled folks.

I generally give away partial scholarship to the majority of people attending my programs. I find that providing more partial scholarships is a better way to spread the benefit instead of a few full scholarships for a few people. Another way to approach this is to find funding to support scholarships, but that can be challenging if you're not a nonprofit. Most foundations or grant-giving organizations want to give directly to a nonprofit. If you are considering organizing a nonprofit, you can start by finding a fiscal sponsor, which is another nonprofit that acts as an umbrella organization for you.[50]

Yet another way to make your offerings financially accessible is to look for third-party funders. For example, you could have a class at a hospital and try to get the hospital to pay you through their wellness program, or you could work with an organization that serves disabled people, older adults, or youth, and see if they'll support you. That's the way I taught for most of my career. I offered my classes in hospitals and through organizations like the National Multiple Sclerosis Society.

The benefit of this structure is that the organization would pay me directly, and then the students would either make a small donation back to the organization, or come for free. It shifted the dynamic of the class tremendously, both in obvious and subtle ways. One obvious change was that my student base became much more diverse. I had many people coming to class who I had never seen in my traditional studio classes, which was very exciting.

On the less obvious side, I could feel a shift in my relationship with the students because I was no longer looking to them to pay me. Also, I was being paid a flat rate, and so it wouldn't matter if there were two students or twenty. I didn't need a bigger group to make more money, and that changed the way I thought about class attendance.

Financial Ethics

Of course there's a bigger question here: If you're not of South Asian descent, is it okay to be making money from teaching yoga, or is it a form of appropriation to make money from this indigenous practice? I personally think it's okay for yoga teachers to get paid because we have to survive as well, and we are providing a valuable service. But we need to be giving back in some way.

Can you support marginalized communities with your time and energy, or literally offer some form of financial reparations? It's also essential to consider whether your pricing is fair, reasonable, and is helping to make the practice more accessible to others. In general, I believe that yoga is free and people are paying for my basic needs so I can have housing and food for myself and my family. They're not really paying for the yoga.

I also need to make sure that I'm practicing yoga in all my interactions, so any business practices need to reflect yoga's ethical teachings, such as non-greed and non-hoarding. I also think it's fine to teach for free if you have another job or another source of income.

In fact, there are times when it's important to do so, especially when it's an act of giving back.

Teaching for free on occasion is also an effective way to reach more people in the form of marketing. When I was first starting out, I would often teach the first class for free, whether I was approaching a new organization or a support group. I would tell them I can teach one class for free so your community can see if that is a practice that would be helpful for them.

A slightly controversial way of making yoga accessible is through work exchange programs. When I was younger, I took a lot of yoga classes this way, by working reception desks in exchange for classes. While I do think there are some benefits to these arrangements and to bartering in general, I also think there are a lot of potential dangers here as well. First of all, this isn't karma yoga, even though it's often referred to as such.

Karma yoga is service offered out of love. Work exchange is bartering. Work exchange agreements need to be explicit and fair, and there needs to be an understanding that work exchange is still a form of employment, and the people doing the work must be treated fairly. This also applies to volunteers. Additionally, it's important to be aware of tax laws around work exchange.

Recently, there was news of a large yoga chain, Yoga to the People, that used some of these practices—work exchange and by-donation classes—to launder money. Not only did they avoid paying taxes, they also didn't pay their employees.[51] This is a perfect example of how these seemingly progressive financial ideas may be used not only in the mission of service, but also for selfishness and greed.

Accessible Spaces

When most people think of accessibility they think of wheelchair users and questions of physical accessibility: Are the doors wide enough for a wheelchair? Do the doors open easily enough? Are the bathrooms spacious enough? Etc. But there are many other factors to consider when making a physical space accessible.

One issue I always notice is that people tend to leave their shoes around the door of yoga studios. Piles of shoes can make it impossible for a wheelchair to pass through easily. Also, is there a ramp or elevator to get into the building, and is the furniture laid out in the lobby or waiting area easy to navigate around?

Additional concerns include the use of incense or highly scented products which may make a space inaccessible for someone with chemical sensitivity. Are there sufficient yoga props, and are they being used during class? Is there a therapy bed, or a raised platform where a wheelchair user could more easily transfer to a horizontal surface?

If you really want to make your offerings accessible to disabled people, it's important to take a holistic approach. Consider universal design, which is a practice of designing the environment for all people. It's about making change within society to fit our lives rather than the other way around. So universal design would be understanding all the factors that would potentially interfere with someone coming to a yoga class. It could be someone's busy schedule, their inability to find public transportation to the class location, the pricing structure, the way the room is set up, etc.

Labeling Your Classes

I've always said, "Outer ability ≠ inner peace!" In fact, we used to print that slogan on our Accessible Yoga t-shirts. Sure, it's great to be strong and flexible, but that's not the goal of yoga. Physical ability is not a reflection of how advanced your yoga practice is. If it were, what would happen when you get older and can't do the same poses anymore?

My grandmother practiced yoga into her 80s, and slowly could do less and less. She wasn't becoming more of a beginner. We've gotten confused. It might be best to simply move away from using terms like "beginner" or "advanced" to describe yoga practice, since it just leads to confusion. We need to find new terminology to describe the practices we are leading.

I appreciate terms like, "all levels," or "mixed levels," but are we truly able to serve all students who come to the class? In my conversation with Tristan Katz for this chapter, that is what they spoke to so clearly: Labels can be misleading and even dangerous. It might be more effective to consider describing the content or focus of a class rather than the level of physical ability.

For example, rather than "beginner" or "advanced" you could give your classes titles that speak to their content, such as, Yoga for Relaxation, Yoga for Strength, or Yoga for Flexibility. Otherwise, we're continuing to perpetuate an ableist narrative that is at odds with yoga's fundamental philosophy that we are all equal in spirit.

Affinity Classes

Most of the time, in Accessible Yoga, we're focusing on how to serve the broadest spectrum of students possible within one yoga class. But there's also an opportunity to create what we call affinity spaces or specialty classes for a specific group of people who want to be together or that you want to teach separately from others.

Affinity groups in general are a great way for groups that experience marginalization to build community and to be in a safe space. In these spaces, they may be able to avoid some of the systemic issues that come up when they're dealing with the larger culture. So there is a great benefit in providing classes for specific populations.

Classes can be specialized because of gender identity, race, disability, or even religion. There are many reasons why you might want to teach a specific group, and I've definitely done this a lot around disability. I've taught special classes for people with HIV/AIDS, heart disease, multiple sclerosis, and other disabilities.

I find there's tremendous potential in these classes, because there's a shared connection among the students. You can teach in a way that emphasizes that connection and community building, and you also want to make sure to design a class based on the needs of the participants.

Sometimes these special classes aren't based on bringing together a specific group of people, rather they are based on serving a group of people in a particular location. For example, teaching yoga in a prison, a school, a residential treatment center, or an older adult living facility. Many of the same considerations arise for these classes as for other specialty classes.

Whether you want to teach a yoga class for people with larger bodies at a yoga studio or teach a yoga class in a county jail, in order for your offering to be effective, you first need to consider why you want to teach this particular community. Do you have a personal connection? Or, is it rooted in a white savior complex? According to Anti-Racism Daily, which was founded by yoga teacher, Nicole Cardoza:

The term white savior complex refers to the belief that white people have a responsibility or a right to save or rescue people of color from their problems or circumstances. The white savior complex often involves a sense of superiority and a lack of awareness of one's own privilege, and it can manifest in a variety of ways, including charitable or philanthropic efforts, missionary work, or intervention in social or political issues.

The white savior complex can have harmful consequences, including perpetuating harmful stereotypes, undermining the agency and self-determination of people of color, and contributing to a culture of paternalism and dependency. Some critics argue that the white savior complex represents a form of colonialism or neocolonialism, in which white people attempt to impose their own solutions or values on people of color without fully understanding or respecting their cultures or experiences.[52]

One way to avoid the white savior complex is to ask yourself if you do actually have a personal connection with the group you want to serve. If not, it might be better to share resources with that community, to lift up members from that community directly. You could even train people within that community to be yoga teachers themselves so that you don't have to do it.

In fact, Accessible Yoga started in 2007 because I wanted to train my disabled students to become yoga teachers. For years, I had been encouraging many of them to take teacher training, but they felt that most programs were not accessible to them. So we started an Accessible Yoga Teacher Training and many of them became teachers.

Collaboration

Once you've done some reflection and decided on a community that you want to teach, you can begin to look around and see who is already serving that community. For example, if you think, "I would love to teach yoga for people with cancer." There are many teachers and organizations already doing that. So rather than starting your own new yoga for cancer organization, why not look at what already exists and see if you can work with them, support them, or collaborate with them in some way?

I feel like collaboration is a lost art. Perhaps it's an outcome of the individualism in our society. Personally, I have found that collaborating with other like-minded people to build something together has been the greatest experience of my life. Accessible Yoga is built on collaboration and connection. At all our conferences I challenge all the attendees to find someone else at the program that they can collaborate with or elevate in some way.

So do some research and find out who's already serving the community you want to reach. Then, using your networking skills, reach out to them and see what possibilities might exist. When you are networking, it's important to approach people with offers of support. I've often had people approach me asking for something. They might email me and say, "I have this new project, can you help me with it?" As much as I want to support all yoga teachers, I've also learned that I have limited resources. So I find it's more effective if someone who is interested in my work asks how they can learn from me or work with me—rather than trying to get me to work for them.

Networking is an essential skill for yoga teachers. I think I got all my teaching jobs that way. I would start by assisting a teacher who was doing work I was interested in, and offer to sub for them. Or, I would take a training or workshop with them and follow up and say how much I love the work they're doing, and that I'm looking for teaching opportunities in that area.

Designing Specialty Classes

When it comes to actually teaching yoga to special populations it's important to take the time to do the research and training required. Of course, the first step is to ask the students directly: What are the things your community needs? Do you need strengthening practices or nervous system regulation, and relaxation? Do you need inspiration and uplifting spiritual teachings, community building and a sense of belonging, or even fun?

You can also consider specific contraindications for this community. Are there practices that might be dangerous or exacerbate a condition? With the example of yoga for cancer, it's important to do some research or special training.[53] Many people with cancer end up with osteoporosis as a result of chemotherapy, so you need to think about what that means for a yoga class. You'd want to be extra careful about students falling, and support them in gently building strength and bone density.

You may need specialized training when working with some communities such as incarcerated populations, veterans, or survivors of abuse. Remember that those communities have experienced specific trauma that needs special considerations. When teaching them you may need to avoid specific poses or language, which I'll cover more in detail in chapter eleven. Generally, spend time researching what would be least harmful and most beneficial to your community, as well as how to best reach them.

There are many other communities that benefit from specialized classes. You can design classes for neurodiverse students, refugees, immigrants, the Blind/low vision community, communities of color, the queer and Trans community, and so many more. These classes may take special skills, such as serving the Deaf/deaf and hard of hearing community, where you may need to speak sign language and have familiarity with Deaf culture. The possibilities are endless, and give an opportunity for creativity and collaboration.

Teaching in Special Locations

To reach specific populations, it is often necessary to bring yoga to them. Consider starting classes where your community is already gathering. It can be a lot more effective than starting a class in a local studio and waiting for people to come to you. Of course, when you teach in the community there are a number of factors to consider. You are probably teaching in a space that isn't designed for yoga, so you'll have to do the extra work of holding a strong container for the group.

What often happens if you're teaching in a gym, school, hospital, prison, community center, or outside, is that there may be multiple distractions and noises going on around you. There may be people wandering in and out of your space as well. The first thing is to make sure that all your students can hear you and see you, and then do your best to keep them focused. Sometimes this means acknowledging the disturbances and using them as a part of the practice.

One hospital where I taught had an announcement system that couldn't be turned off. We were practicing in a conference room, and every once in a while we would hear, "Code blue! Code blue!" which meant that someone was having a life-threatening emergency. It would often happen when we were in *shavasana* or meditation, and I tried many different ways to integrate it into the class. I finally realized that we couldn't ignore these announcements. We needed to pause what we were doing, and send prayers to whoever was struggling in the ER. Over the years, I found that those interruptions actually became a powerful reminder of our mortality, and the power of prayer.

The other issue with teaching outside of traditional studio settings is that you have to handle the registration process yourself, which includes having students sign waivers, make payments, and sign in for class. In this case, it's helpful to create efficient systems ahead of time and try to have students complete as much of that process as possible before arriving.

Also, you either have to carry around lots of props, find a way to store props in that location, or teach without props. Personally, I find that chair yoga is especially effective in many of these settings because chairs are almost always present, and there are endless practices that can be experienced in a chair. Walls are also a really useful prop for many practices. Students can lean against a wall in seated poses, stand with their back to a wall in balancing poses, practice legs up the wall, and so much more.

Liability Insurance & Waivers

In the U.S., I always recommend that yoga teachers have liability insurance and have all their students sign waivers[54] before participating in class. These relatively simple steps can help to protect you legally, and also provide students with additional information. Waivers can include general contraindications for asana practice and help to remind students that they are responsible for their well-being in class.

I had a yoga teacher friend who was sued by a student after they were injured in her class. The judge said that the waiver was proof that the student understood the risks of practicing yoga, and found that the teacher wasn't liable. Of course, I'm not a lawyer, so I recommend getting legal advice if you are concerned about this.

Scenario

Imagine that you're teaching a series of classes, and you have policies stated clearly on your website where people sign up, including a refund policy that says no refunds are allowed once the program begins. After the first session a student emails you and says, "I don't have time to complete this course. Can I get a refund?" How do you respond?

Response

This is a situation that I come across pretty often. I understand that people have busy lives and tend to not read policies when signing up for things. To me, part of ethical practice is following through on the rules I create for my community. If I don't follow through on my policies, it shows that they aren't important to me.

This could mean that I need to update or change my policies to reflect how I truly feel.

At the same time, I like to be a compassionate person, and I understand that people sometimes have emergencies, or that their financial situation can change very quickly. For this reason, I do always consider what the person is saying when they ask for a refund. If it is an emergency, I do consider a partial or full refund depending on how far along we are in the course. Another option is to offer the student a credit toward a future program rather than a refund.

I've recently added language to my refund policy that individual situations will be considered, so that I can take these situations into account and still feel that I'm following the ethical guidelines I created for myself.

Further Reflection

- Consider whether your efforts to create accessible and welcoming spaces could potentially backfire, and if there is something you can do to ensure it doesn't?

- Do you have a pricing policy that is reflective of your understanding and practice of yoga?

- Are the spaces you teach in physically accessible? Can you take it one step further and consider universal design, where the environment is created with accessibility in mind?

- How do you label your classes?

- Are there specific communities you want to reach with yoga, and why?

- If you're teaching yoga outside of a studio, what could you do to make those classes even more accessible and effective?

CHAPTER SEVEN

MAKING YOGA ACCESSIBLE

As far as the yoga tradition is concerned, postures and tech-niques aren't end goals in and of themselves. Instead they are tools. I try to start people with, "Put your hand here. Let's feel how that feels. Put your hand there. Let's feel how that feels." In an example like this, I'm offering two options which are both mechanically similar. If neither works, we keep experimenting to land on the one that fits.

In pretty much every class, I really try to expose people to two to three different ways of working on at least two to three different poses. There's almost never a singular way to practice a pose that we're exploring in depth. There's a range, and you have to play within this range and figure out which one doesn't work, and which one does work best for you.

When I give you cues, if those cues don't make you feel better and more equanimous in the pose, then they're not good cues for you. They're just me doing my best, but I'm not more of an authority than you are. Perhaps I'd be more of an author-ity if we were just drawing pretty pictures with a body that had limitless options, and we were trying to recreate the images in Light on Yoga, *but your sensory experience is greater than my visual understanding of what I'm seeing in your body. So I'm giving you a range and letting you know that even when I*

123

cue you, I might be wrong. I have a more distant assessment of your experience than you do. So I'm going to give you my thoughts, but they're just meant to help you. If they don't help you then get rid of them.

As a teacher, when people are coming to your public classes and they need a more adaptable environment, do your best. Be nice. Bust out some props for them. Be inclusive in a way that lets people normalize the challenges that often arise in yoga class. Instead of giving limited options and making yoga class into a small little exclusive world, just relate to people. Look them in their eyes. Be nice. Say, "I'm glad you're here."

—Jason Crandell

WHEN I INTERVIEWED Jason Crandell for this book, he started out the interview by saying he didn't know why I wanted to interview him on a topic I'm more knowledgeable about. While I appreciate his faith in me, I also recognize that he is an extremely experienced and established teacher who is well respected for his clear and concise technique. Mostly, I was interested in hearing a slightly more mainstream approach to a topic that I am completely absorbed in, and I learned a lot.

From that conversation, I realized that there's still a clear divide in the yoga world between "traditional" yoga, and Accessible Yoga. People think that teaching Accessible Yoga is some kind of specialty or niche. But that's a false divide. There is really just yoga and the many multifaceted ways that we attempt to share it.

So much of what Jason described about his approach to teaching connects directly to my experience. In particular, I appreciated when he spoke about the importance of a yoga teacher having the right attitude when teaching a mixed-level group, and that it's truly the most advanced form of teaching. He also said that if you don't know how to teach someone how to experience a pose, don't just have them lie in shavasana. Try to find a way in for them, and remember, collaboration is the key.

Jason also talked about how the goal of asana is to create an equanimous experience in the body—a sense of awareness equally distributed, rather than a lot of sensation in any one area. Even if one part of the body is working harder than the others, you don't lose track of everything else. Otherwise, there may be straining or potentially injury. This seems like useful guidance for newer students who may be straining to perform an asana, rather than focusing on their inward experience.

When teaching asana, it's important to ask yourself what makes a physical posture or movement yoga? Is it because it's a traditional shape that has been passed down from ancient yogis, or is it because of an internal process that's occurring while your body is making a specific shape or moving in a particular way?

Reflection

What makes a movement or a position an asana?

Six Steps toward Accessibility

Honestly, it hurts my heart to think of all the people who avoid yoga, or worse, have negative experiences in yoga, because they think it's all about being flexible, strong, and agile. If only they could see that yoga is about coming home to yourself, and that yoga is a practice for everyone.

I wonder how we got to this point? I guess it's a combination of factors: A competitive industry with lots of money at stake, a colonizer mindset always looking to brand something, and our generally competitive nature. The truth of yoga often isn't shared or taught because it's about giving people agency over their own bodies and lives. It's about empowering people to be truly independent, and that kind of independence might not be good for business! You have an essential role in changing this dynamic. Here are six tips for moving toward greater accessibility in your classes. I've touched on most of these points already, and I'll cover the others in the rest of the book:

1. Focus on universal teachings
2. Keep students safe
3. Adapt practices
4. Provide choices
5. Teach truly mixed-level classes
6. Destigmatize chair and bed yoga

Teaching Chair Yoga

I'm a big proponent of chair yoga, and I spend a lot of my time trying to show students how you can get the same benefits of yoga from chair practice. One of the biggest hurdles that I see to practicing in a chair is this false idea that if you're not doing asana on a yoga mat on the floor then you're not really doing yoga. It's such a shame, because it really prevents people from practicing. I've even had students who simply refuse to practice in a chair, even though it would be safer for them. (By the way, if that happens I usually have the whole class practice in a chair.)

There are a few things to consider when teaching chair yoga to help keep students safe. One is to make sure that the chair is sturdy. I've had chairs break while students were practicing in them, and that was dangerous and upsetting. Also, make sure that your students won't fall out of their chairs by avoiding quick forward movements and considering having them keep one foot on the floor at all times.

The other thing to keep in mind about chair yoga is that the students aren't starting from a neutral anatomical position. Their hips and knees are in flexion, which can impact any movements. Sitting for long periods of time may be associated with increased posterior pelvic tilt or a slouching posture.[55] So it's important to consider whether additional spinal flexion (rounding the back) is useful.

Also, the bottom of the pelvis is the main grounding point in chair yoga. That means that the body weight is on the pelvis which makes the pelvis more stable and less mobile than if you're practicing standing or even lying down. In some chair yoga poses, a fixed pelvis could create more stress on the lower back or sacroiliac joints, so try to be conscious of that when teaching. This is especially true of twists and forward bends, as well as asymmetrical poses like triangle pose where it's important to move the pelvis and spine in a unified way.

There are also so many potential benefits to chair yoga. It offers an accessible format for almost everyone, including students who could practice on the floor. Chair yoga can be done at the office, in an airplane, or anywhere there are chairs. Chair yoga can also be combined with standing/wall work, or bed yoga, to create a powerful practice. For example, an effective combination of chair and bed practice is to do some chair yoga sitting on a couch, and then recline on the couch for shavasana or other supine poses.

When teaching chair yoga, very little needs to change about your class other than the orientation that students are practicing from. So, if you're new to the practice, try doing some chair yoga yourself, and get a feel for what works for your body.

Of course, there are some elements that may be lost in chair yoga such as the physical massage that lying on the floor creates. So you can recreate that massage with props, like using a bolster on your lap in cobra pose, *bhujangasana*, and allowing the abdomen to gently press into the bolster as you bend forward.

Another element that may be lost in chair yoga is the strengthening aspect of many asanas when done on the mat. To make up for this, it may be helpful to add specific strengthening practices such as isometric exercises, where the muscles contract without movement. These can be done with the upper and lower body, and I include many examples in my book, *Accessible Yoga: Poses and Practices for Every Body*.

With experience, I think you'll find that chair yoga provides freedom, accessibility, and an opportunity for deep practice for so many people who thought that yoga was not for them.

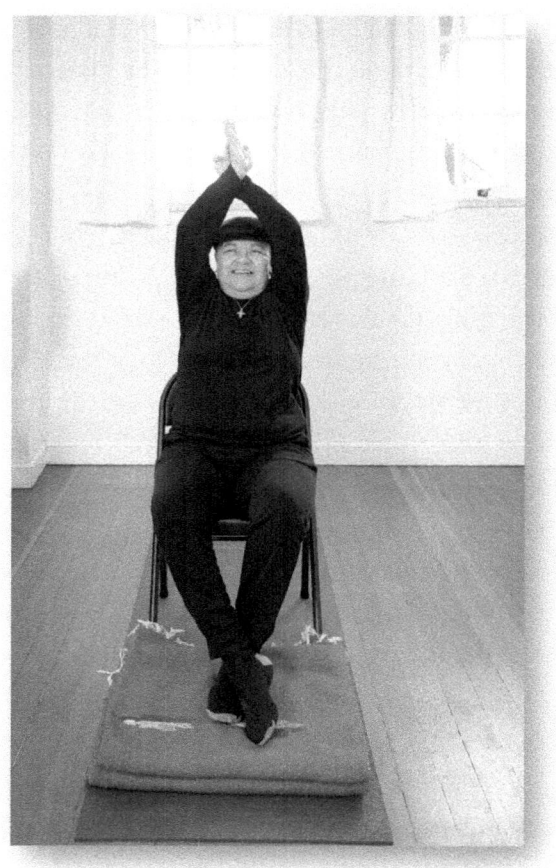

Chair variation of eagle pose, garudasana.

Teaching Bed Yoga

Bed yoga is such a beautiful practice for anyone who wants to experience yoga reclined. This includes people with mobility challenges, older adults, those pre- or post-surgery, and anyone who feels like it. Many people practice in bed before they go to sleep or when they wake up in the morning.

The main thing about bed yoga is that you're practicing on a very different surface than a yoga mat on a hardwood floor. Beds are generally very soft and provide little resistance, or something to push against. This lack of resistance can actually make asana practice more challenging in a way. To create a little more resistance, you could take the blankets off the bed and place a yoga mat on the mattress.

Because it's such a different surface to practice from, it's important to get experience practicing in bed yourself before teaching it. Notice what poses are comfortable and which ones feel awkward. Generally, I only teach supine and side lying poses, since those feel safest. Definitely no standing poses or headstands! (Well, I do teach a bed handstand where the student raises their hands overhead and presses them into the headboard).

You can teach restorative yoga practices in bed, but you don't need to limit yourself to those. Bed yoga can include dynamic movement, strengthening, and flexibility. As with anything you're teaching, consider what your student's individual needs are and design a practice that is going to be most helpful for them. Bed yoga is generally taught one-on-one, so there is more opportunity to personalize the practice.

Standing poses work well in bed yoga by using the footboard of the bed as the floor. You can also make creative use of the props at hand, including bed pillows, towels, and blankets. A hospital bed where you can raise the head or the feet provides many additional options.

Interoception & Proprioception

Interoception is the sense of what is happening inside the body. Increased interoception is one of the most important benefits of yoga practice. In my mind, it may actually be the mark of an experienced practitioner. Interoception is the recognition of inner sensations such as the breath, heartbeat, hunger, and energy moving in the body.

Many disabled people and those with chronic illness—in particular, chronic pain—already have increased sensitivity and an increased understanding of their body's signals and inner life. Therefore, they already have increased interceptive abilities. So for these practitioners, there may be other goals to work on, such as increased strength, or stress reduction, or the larger spiritual goals of the practice.

Another important general benefit of asana practice is increased proprioception. Proprioception is the ability to know where your body is in space and what it's doing without looking at it with your eyes. In order to move the body into different shapes, students first need to know where their body is.

Notice if students are having challenges with proprioception, or if the issue is mobility. Sometimes the messages aren't getting through the nervous system and sometimes there is another reason why a body doesn't respond, such as injury or paralysis. Knowing the cause may help the student figure out the most effective way to practice.

One of the issues that comes up quite often is an imbalance between two sides of the body. For example, after a stroke, it's very common that one side of the body is extremely limited, while the other side may have a full range of motion. In this case, the question is whether the side that is limited should be moved to create some balance or symmetry.

On the one hand, I see that there is potential benefit in assisting the more limited side to move, but to me that also feels more like physical therapy. Not being able to move the limited side might feel frustrating for the student, so that might not be ideal either. There's also a third option, which is practicing mentally. Visualizing practice is very powerful, and it takes a good amount of concentration. The student can lift the more mobile arm, and imagine the limited side moving in a similar way. In the end, I would consider which way of practicing brings more peace and calm, and go with that. I would also be sure to work within my scope of practice, and be sure to have consent if touch is involved.

It may be helpful to spend time working on proprioception without movement, or with small movements. For example, an opening centering practice can be an exploration of sensations in the body, focusing on sensing physical and energetic cues about the body. Students can note the sense of grounding where their body is touching the floor, chair, or other props. They can explore the feeling of their clothes against their skin, and the temperature of the air. Then they can find the center of gravity in the body, rocking from side to side or back and forth, or in small circles. It can also be helpful to imagine drawing the outline of the body with the mind to create a mental image of the body in space.

Of course, balancing poses are a great way to explore proprioception, and there are many ways to make them more accessible. Eagle pose is one of my favorite poses, and students can practice standing with their back to a wall, so they can feel fully supported and strong. Eagle also works well in a chair. To focus on balance in the chair version, you can shift the body weight forward and explore finding your center of gravity. Any conscious physical practice helps students increase their interoception and proprioception and can lead to increased steadiness and comfort, which are the defining elements of asana.

Online Teaching

Online teaching creates both benefits and challenges for yoga teachers and students. For students, the benefits to practicing online include increased accessibility, choice of teachers and styles of classes, ease of scheduling, and often less expense. Online, students can often find a community that feels truly aligned with their personal needs because there are so many options out there.

Practicing online usually means being at home, which may feel like a safer environment than a studio with a group of people they may not know. This sense of safety may allow students to go deeper and can be very effective for people who have experienced trauma. An online practice can encourage students to pay more attention to their inner experience and focus inwardly. In-person classes may bring out their competitive side and encourage them to focus on what other people are doing. So online practice may be particularly helpful for those who have a competitive nature.

Technology itself may be either a blessing or a barrier when it comes to accessing online teaching. For some, access to a computer with fast internet speed may be challenging, and for others, options like closed captioning make online classes more accessible.

In terms of making yoga safe and accessible, sharing online classes may be the right choice depending on the community you're hoping to reach. At the same time, there are benefits to practicing in person that may be lost. In online classes, it can take more effort for students to connect with each other and benefit from the social aspect of an in-person class.

For this reason, it can be incredibly useful to make a concerted effort to increase the community aspect of your online classes. You could do this by spending time having students introduce themselves or doing some sharing at the beginning of class. Or, save some time at the end of class for talking or answering questions the way you might in person.

Online teaching creates a few additional unique challenges for teachers: Do you focus on watching the students or focus on demonstrating the practices that you're teaching? As I discuss in the section on demonstrating on page 150, there is tremendous power in it for students who are visual learners, Deaf/deaf and hard of hearing, or who aren't fluent in whatever language you're teaching in. Even for students who don't fit into those categories, demonstrating practices can be encouraging and helpful when they are newer to the practice and just learning how to connect with their bodies.

So, if you're doing a lot of demonstrating, chances are you're not able to spend a lot of time watching what the students are doing. This isn't that different from demonstrating in person, but it seems even more challenging when teaching online. I know some teachers who create a special setup just to address this situation. They have a second, large monitor where they display the students' videos. Some teachers hook up a television for this so they can watch it while they're back on their mat or chair demoing.

Another challenge of teaching online is being able to get useful feedback from the way the students are moving or responding to your cues. In person, it can be easy to see someone's hesitation or reaction to something we say. You might hear them breathing heavily, or holding their breath, or you can get a reading on their energy level or emotional state. Online it can be harder to have that level of awareness, especially if someone is muted or their video is turned off. In the end, online teaching offers a great option for many people and communities that may not otherwise have access to yoga, but it's not the right medium for everyone.

When teaching online it's important that the students can see and hear you easily. So it's helpful to invest in your setup, not just financially, but also by putting the time in to set up your teaching space and test out your equipment. If you're demonstrating, it can be helpful to wear a lavalier mic rather than relying on the mic on your computer. That way the sound won't be compromised when you're far away from the computer.

In order for students to easily see you, it can be helpful to invest in some adjustable lighting and set up your space so that you have a clean, neutral background. Also, check your camera angle and distance so that students can see your entire body when you're demonstrating. Wearing solid, dark colors against a light background also helps make it easier for students to see you. Recording yourself teaching and then watching it back is an effective way to check on your sound and video quality so that you can offer the most effective online teaching experience possible.

Intake Process

An Accessible Yoga class is an opportunity to address the needs of each individual within a group setting. This can be a challenge for a teacher if the class is large, so consider having assistants in class if you have more students than you can safely support on your own. Assistants can be newer yoga teachers looking for experience, or a peer with whom you take turns assisting at each other's classes.

It's helpful to have enough information about each student to keep them safe, so you may want to implement some form of intake process. For yoga teachers, this can be very simple. Before beginning class, it's important to connect with each student individually. This can be done through a registration form, a verbal intake, or if you are practicing yoga therapy, it can be a more detailed written intake. In person this can be done by arriving early and checking in with each student as they arrive. The same can be done online, but there is even less privacy in an online class, and students may be less willing to share.

There is another subtler aspect to doing some form of intake, and that is simply getting to know your students better. Not only does this help to create community, but it can give you clues regarding the content of your classes. For example, if a few students talk about feeling extra tired, it might be nice to teach a more relaxed class. Or, if someone complains of having a sore neck, you could add in some additional neck stretches. Also, an intake gives you a chance to find out the students' intentions for coming to yoga. Are they looking for relaxation, physical healing, strengthening, flexibility, or spiritual awakening?

Addressing the needs of each individual student is one of the benefits of teaching an integrated mixed-level Accessible Yoga class. In an integrated class, different levels of a pose can be practiced simultaneously, and each student is actively engaged. What we want to avoid is having one student "sit out" of a pose because we can't figure out a variation that is appropriate. I'll discuss how to teach integrated classes in the next chapter.

It is not within the scope of practice of yoga teachers to ask students for medical information. But there are some useful questions you can ask in a simple intake, including:

- Have you done yoga before? If so, how was it?
- If not, do you do other forms of exercise or movement?
- Is there anything going on with your body today that you want me to know about that will help me keep you safe during the class?
- Do you want to practice in a chair or on a mat?

Also, just because you don't ask for medical information doesn't mean that someone won't volunteer it. If someone reports having recent surgery or an injury, it can be helpful to ask if their healthcare provider has approved them for exercise. Even though a yoga class isn't an exercise class, that is the terminology that medical providers use to say whether or not it's safe for someone to participate in any kind of movement practice. If there is any confusion about this, you can always provide information about what kinds of poses and practices you'll be doing in class so that the student has specific information to ask their provider about.

One-on-One Teaching

One-on-one private instruction is not always accessible because of financial reasons. Yet, most people would greatly benefit from it, whether they are new to yoga and have lots of questions, or because they need more individualized direction or support. Some tips for leading private sessions include:

- Find out the student's intention for wanting a private session so you can serve them to the best of your ability.
- Be clear about your scope of practice (which I discussed at length in chapter two) and what areas you can confidently support them with.
- Be sure to conduct an appropriate intake and assessment to better understand the student's needs and goals for your time together. The details of this intake will depend on your scope of practice.
- Keep notes of your work together so you can track your student's progress, as well as build on their successes.
- Consider assigning homework that will help empower the student and help them work toward building a personal home practice.
- Consider the setup of the room you're teaching in. Sometimes, one-on-one students benefit from practicing alongside the teacher, as a co-practice, rather than having the teacher facing them the entire time, which can be intimidating. This might feel different online, so experiment with different set ups for one-on-one classes you're teaching virtually.
- When teaching a student who is practicing in a bed, be sure to take care of your own body, especially if you plan to assist the student's movement during the session. You may need to demonstrate from a standing or seated position so they can see what you're doing—you definitely don't want to lie next to them in bed!

Inspiring Home Practice

The sign of a successful yoga teacher is empowered students who embrace their own practice and make yoga an important part of their lives. A home practice is the most effective way to dive deep into the teachings and practice of yoga, and if handled well, class time can be a gateway to a regular personal practice.

A few ways to inspire home practice include:

- Have a strong personal practice of your own, and talk about it with your students. (By the way, a strong practice doesn't mean you don't have your own struggles, or that you practice every single day, but that you are committed to it in the long run.)
- Talk about the importance and benefits of regular practice.
- Offer tips for starting home practice, such as creating a special space in your home, and finding a regular time to practice each day.
- Give students homework, such as, "Practice your favorite pose every day this week," or "Try to practice five minutes of yoga each day this week."
- Follow up on homework and ask students how they felt practicing a little each day.

Class Planning

Teaching yoga is a combination of good planning and spontaneous creativity. Being well prepared with a clear class plan is essential, but it's also important to be able to adapt to the students in front of you and be willing to change that plan in the moment. I plan all my classes and then usually let go of that plan when I see or feel that something different is needed.

A class plan can look like a simple outline of practices. In my mind, there is nothing wrong with coming to class with a written outline of what you propose to teach. Rather than showing a lack of preparedness, I think it actually shows the opposite—that you care enough to plan ahead.

When creating a plan, you need to consider the overarching goals of the class and the needs of the students. Often new teachers want to give everything they know all at once and in every class. It's important to pace yourself and not overwhelm your students with information.

Most of all, it's important to model the teachings of yoga in the way you teach and in how you treat the students. In the end what students will take away from your class is an experience and a feeling that they found there. Over time the details will fade away, but the feeling you gave them will remain. There's a famous quote from Dr. Maya Angelou about this. She said:

> *People will forget what you said, people will forget what you did, but people will never forget how you made them feel.*[56]

In terms of creating long-term impact, it may be more effective to share a regular sequence that you repeat in each class. Or, at least a very similar structure that students can come to expect. This may be calming to your students and is considered trauma-informed. Of course, many students want something new each time, and I see lots of yoga teachers constantly looking to add something interesting or new to their classes. But, I wonder if it's really necessary? There is nothing new about yoga, and there is a reason it has withstood the test of time.

Also, there is a misunderstanding that Accessible Yoga is always gentle. My goal is to share a practice that supports my students in their life goals. If their goal is to be stronger and more fit, then we can find a way to address that in our classes. In fact, I generally think more physical activity is good for our bodies and our minds.

The challenge is often finding a physically intense practice that doesn't cause injury, especially if someone has a preexisting condition such as a back problem (which includes about half of all older adults[57]). An interesting example is working with people with arthritis.[58] Most osteoarthritis improves with movement, but it can be painful. It's difficult to know whether we should encourage students to push through the pain, or use the pain as a signal to stop or slow down.

This is an even bigger challenge for students with chronic pain. How do they know how far to push themselves in physical practice if the cue of stopping when you feel pain loses meaning? One thing I've found over the years is that these students often won't know until after class, or even the next day, whether they pushed themselves too far. I ask them to notice how well they sleep that night, and how they feel the next day. If they have increased pain then they may have pushed themselves too far.

Reflection

Do you feel pressure to create fancy choreography to keep your students interested, or can you focus on the heart of the practice?

Sequencing & Pacing

Specific pose sequences are often taught by various yoga lineages in an effort to brand a series of practices. In fact, years ago, Bikram tried and failed to copyright his class series in what felt like an effort to further commodify modern yoga.[59] It's not necessary to follow a specific set sequence to teach an effective class, but there are important things to keep in mind. In the end, common sense is the most important element when it comes to sequencing.

I always recommend opening and closing classes with centering practices. These are subtle practices to bookend the class and expose students to the power of yoga. (I'll discuss subtle practices in detail in part three.) During the movement, or asana, section, consider how you will warm up and prepare before teaching any challenging poses. Try to include all the movements of the spine—often a simple combination of backward and forward bending, side-bending, gentle inversions, and twists build a wonderful class.

Consider the pacing and length of class. Sometimes less is more, and rather than wear out your students, leave them energized and relaxed at the same time—an experience many people are completely unfamiliar with.

You also need to think about how much time you spend in each asana. Repeating a pose a few times for shorter periods of time can be more accessible to many people than holding a static pose for longer. Plus, there is some debate about the benefits and risks of static stretching. Some research seems to show that it may decrease performance in athletes.[60] At the same time, older adults may benefit from static stretching.[61]

Dynamic practice, coming in and out of a pose with the breath, is a good way to stretch without doing static stretching. Over time, you can take cues from your students to find out how long to be in a pose or how long the whole class should be. Find the balance of challenge, fun, and relaxation.

Remember that what works for your body, or for some students, may not work for others. So, how do you find the proper balance? If a longer class is useful for most students, but there are a few who get exhausted from it, what do you do? These types of challenges come up in every group class.

To me, the answer lies in creating an atmosphere of acceptance and inner listening. I would hope that if one of my students felt tired, that they had the personal agency to stop practicing and rest, regardless of what everyone else was doing. I recommend you try it some time. Doing nothing while other people practice around you is a very interesting and challenging practice for your mind.

When planning an Accessible Yoga class sequence it's helpful to think about practices that can be easily done on the mat and in the chair simultaneously, which I discuss in detail on page 182. You can also build a class from a theme, focusing on the benefits of the practices you want to share. You can build a class that focuses on balance, strength, relaxation/stress reduction, meditation, flexibility/mobility, grounding, energizing, or more. For example, if I was creating a class sequence focused on balance, I might teach something like this:

1. Centering: Meditation on feeling gravity in the body.
2. Warm-ups: Neck, spine, shoulders and hip movements. Spend time working with the feet and ankles to prepare for standing balancing practices, even though not everyone will come to standing.
3. Asana: Integrated practices (that can be done simultaneously on the mat and chair). A backward bend, a forward bend, a twist, and a series of standing balancing poses such as tree, eagle, and king dancer. The focus in these poses would be finding adapted versions that make balancing easier when standing, and practices that challenge balance for people practicing in a chair.
4. Closing Centering: Shavasana, focusing again on working with gravity; a pranayama practice; and a seated meditation with extra time spent finding the center of gravity in the body.

It's also important to consider transitions between orientations such as seated to standing, or lying down to sitting. For many people, these transitions can be one of the most challenging parts of class. This may be because of low or high blood pressure, disability, or age.

Transitions are moments where there is an increased risk of falls for older adults, so if you're teaching that population it's worth sequencing the class in a way that minimizes transitions. This can be done by grouping together practices in different orientations.

For example, if I was teaching a mixed class of older adults, I would start the class with everyone sitting in a chair for centering and warm ups. Then give students an option to come to standing for a series of standing and balancing poses, then move to the floor for some seated or reclined poses, ending in shavasana. Then come back to the chair for final pranayama and meditation. Of course, students would be welcome to stay in the chair for the whole class, and I would focus on creating a smooth flow between poses that prioritizes safety.

In chair yoga, there is a similar, but more simple, flow that I find works very well, especially for online classes where people are at home. We start seated, and then spend some time reclined on a couch or bed, and then come back to seated at the end.

Another way to think about how to sequence a yoga class is to consider the context of the eight limbs of yoga, ashtanga yoga, moving from external to internal. In other words, to teach asana, pranayama, and then meditation. This is also reflected in the *koshas*, moving from the body, to the breath, to the mind, and beyond.

Here's a sample integrated Accessible Yoga class sequence, with some students practicing on a mat and some in chairs:

Check in

- Introduce yourself
- Brief intake—ask each student how they're doing
- Posture check—make sure everyone is in a comfortable position to begin class. In an integrated class everyone could begin sitting in a chair

Opening Centering—could include any of the following:

- Chanting
- Vocalizing
- Pranayama
- Meditation
- Intention-setting

Warm-Ups

- Moving the major joints, neck and spine, shoulders, hips
- Connect movement with breath
- Could be the entire movement portion of the class
- Could include strengthening practices
- Students can stay in the chair or transfer to the mat for these practices

Asana

- Option for some students to stand or come to the mat while some stay in a chair
- Teach in an integrated fashion as described on page 182
- Include a combination of backward and forward bending, gentle inversions, twists, balancing and strengthening poses

Closing Centering—could include any of the following. Students can be on the mat or in the chair:

- Shavasana
- Yoga nidra
- Pranayama
- Meditation

- Dedication, which is offering the benefits of the practice to others or the entire universe

[Note: I included many specific class sequences in my book, *Accessible Yoga: Poses & Practices for Every Body*.]

Teaching Adults

Most of us teach yoga to adults, and adult education is actually quite different than teaching children. In fact, the term, andragogy[62] specifically refers to adult learning, and researcher, Malcolm Knowles, identified these six elements of andragogy:

1. Need to know: Adults need to know the reason for learning something.
2. Foundation: Experience (including error) provides the basis for learning activities.
3. Self-concept: Adults need to be responsible for their decisions on education; involvement in the planning and evaluation of their instruction.
4. Readiness: Adults are most interested in learning subjects having immediate relevance to their work and/or personal lives.
5. Orientation: Adult learning is problem-centered rather than content-oriented.
6. Motivation: Adults respond better to internal versus external motivators[63]

This research speaks to the fact that most adult learners are self-directed, meaning that they need to be in control of their learning process. This point underscores the importance of emphasizing agency and consent within our classes, which I discussed earlier in chapter five.

It's important to remember that many adults haven't been in a learning environment in a long time. They may not remember, or may have lost touch with, the skills needed to learn new things. In particular, they may have lost the ability to translate the words that you're saying into movements in their body. The community of older adults is also an extremely diverse group that includes those who are extremely active as well as those who aren't. There is also an important intersection between older adults and the disability community.[64]

Teaching Disabled Students

The disability community is the largest minority group in the world, made up of well over a billion people.[65] In fact, recent figures show that one in four Americans identify as disabled.[66] Because of the diversity within the disability community it's challenging to come up with specific guidelines for making welcoming spaces, although really this entire book is dedicated to this idea.

It's important to listen to disabled people directly and to learn from them. Rodrigo Souza, a disabled yoga teacher, trains other yoga teachers in working with disabled students. He asks yoga teachers to release ableist assumptions and ideas. In particular, he asks them to let go of the idea of fixing their students, and focus instead of creating a supportive environment:

> *Yoga is not to fix what is broken, but to fall in love with what is broken and change your relationship with it. I fell in love with my broken body and accepted myself as a whole. So hold space for your students, and they will fix themselves. You don't need to fix them.*[67]

Last year, I interviewed my friend and teacher Matthew Sanford for a podcast, and I wanted to share a short quote from that conversation here. Matthew is a disabled yoga teacher who founded the organization Mind Body Solutions. He explains:

> *The fundamental ethic when you're trying to share asana and pranayama with everybody, especially with people with disabilities, is that you have to make them a partner in the grand experiment. Because you can never have enough knowledge when it comes to all these particular conditions. Not only is every one unique just by definition, like snowflakes, but you're never going to erase all of your uncertainty as a teacher by acquiring more and more knowledge. What you're going to do is level the playing field.*
>
> *I'd rather sit shoulder to shoulder with the student rather than across from a student. Because the fire that we're warming our hands at is actually within both of us. I feel like the teachings of yoga have to be shared, they can't really be taught. Usually there's a teacher and student, but my approach is, "Hey, did you feel that? Holy moly. That's awesome." A kind of wandering curiosity leaves room for the student and honors the student, but is also good for the ongoing curiosity of the teacher.*[68]

I also think it's helpful to reflect on the movement for disability justice,[69] and to learn from contemporary disability activists. The term disability justice was coined by Sins Invalid,[70] a collective of disabled queer women of color including Patty Berne, Mia Mingus, and Stacey Milbern. They created a list of ten principles of disability justice:

1. Intersectionality: "We do not live single issue lives"—Audre Lorde. Ableism, coupled with white supremacy, supported by capitalism, underscored by heteropatriarchy, has rendered the vast majority of the world "invalid."

2. Leadership of the Most Impacted: "We are led by those who most know these systems."—Aurora Levins Morales

3. Anti-capitalist Politic: In an economy that sees land and humans as components of profit, we are anti-capitalist by the nature of having non-conforming body/minds.

4. Commitment to Cross-movement Organizing: Shifting how social justice movements understand disability and contextualize ableism, disability justice lends itself to politics of alliance.

5. Recognizing Wholeness: People have inherent worth outside of commodity relations and capitalist notions of productivity. Each person is full of history and life experience.

6. Sustainability: We pace ourselves, individually and collectively, to be sustained long term. Our embodied experiences guide us toward ongoing justice and liberation.

7. Commitment to Cross-disability Solidarity: We honor the insights and participation of all of our community members, knowing that isolation undermines collective liberation.

8. Interdependence: We meet each other's needs as we build toward liberation, knowing that state solutions inevitably extend into further control over lives.

9. Collective Access: As brown, black, and queer-bodied disabled people we bring flexibility and creative nuance that go beyond able-bodied/minded normativity, to be in community with each other.

10. Collective Liberation: No body or mind can be left behind—only moving together can we accomplish the revolution we require.[71]

Teaching Students with Larger Bodies

Many larger bodied students are reclaiming the term "fat," since it's a descriptive term. So awareness of language once again is important.

Practicing yoga in a larger body can be challenging when your teacher doesn't understand how asanas can be adapted (often very easily!) to suit and support your shape. Asanas look different in everyone's bodies, and variations are not one-size-fits-all.

Yoga teacher, Amber Karnes, has been teaching people with larger bodies for many years, and helping to shift our cultural understanding about body size. In a podcast interview that I did with Amber, she described her work:

> *My work is about the journey of self-acceptance which goes hand-in-hand with the yoga practice. I think diet culture is the way that society makes us believe a whole series of things about our bodies. It's this automatic assumption that a thin body is the ultimate ideal and being bigger is bad. We see this manifest in many, many ways in yoga spaces like yoga marketing where we only see thin, able-bodied, hyper-fit, hyper-flexible people.*[72]

She also shares two tips that will allow students with larger bodies to explore yoga more comfortably: Take space and make space.

Take Space: Widen

- Widen the legs to make room for the body in a forward fold.
- Widen the arms if it's uncomfortable to bring the hands together behind the back or overhead (straps make great arm extenders).
- Widen the stance (crawl the right foot toward the right side of the mat and the left foot toward the left) if you're feeling too compressed, if it feels difficult to find your center of gravity, if the posture just doesn't quite feel stable, or if you just appreciate the freedom of a little more space.

Make Space: Move Your Squishy Stuff Out of the Way

- In any pose where the belly is squished against the thigh, reach up and smooth the belly between the legs.
- As you fold forward, use your hands to tuck the low belly up and back toward the pelvis.
- Bring both hands to the inside of the front leg in lunge.
- Tuck the breast/chest tissue under the armpit when reaching across the front of the body.

Teaching Older Adults

Yoga is very popular among older adults, but recent research on yoga injuries showed that older practitioners are much more likely to get hurt than younger practitioners.[73] Also, it may take them longer to bounce back from an injury since our resilience decreases as we age. On the other hand, stamina may actually increase as we age, which means that many older students may have no issues at all with keeping up with a fast-paced class as they age. So with this conflicting information, how do we approach teaching older students?

There is such a large and diverse population of older adults that it can be hard to generalize. But there are a few things that are helpful to keep in mind. One is that many people become hard of hearing as they age. In fact, nearly half of people over seventy-five have hearing loss.[74] This is important to remember as a yoga teacher since so much of our teaching is done through spoken instruction.

Speaking clearly and loudly and projecting your voice is essential. Try not to give a lot of instruction when you face away from students to demonstrate something. Also, you can have some students sit closer to you if they have trouble hearing you.

It's also worth considering whether using music could make it harder for older students or Deaf/deaf and hard of hearing students to follow your instructions. Demonstrating practices can also be incredibly helpful as long as you're clearly demonstrating the practices that you want them to do, and they can easily see you. Even though music can be distracting for students who are hard of hearing, it can be useful to those who have memory loss because music is connected to a part of the brain that is often not affected. So using music is a choice that needs to be made consciously for the students in front of you.

Conditions like arthritis, osteoporosis, and high blood pressure are common among older adults, so it's important to become familiar with common conditions and understand what practices may be contraindicated. For example, doing spinal flexion (forward bending) quickly or with straight legs is generally contraindicated for older adults because of the pervasiveness of osteoporosis and the fact that these movements could potentially lead to bone breaks.[75]

It's important to understand contraindications, and at the same time, we need to be mindful about offering students opportunities to challenge themselves. Finding the balance between stretch and strain, or benefit and injury, is an essential aspect of yoga, especially when working with older adults.

Yoga teacher Sunny Barbee, who teaches yoga to older adults, uses a numeric scale to help her students understand the level of intensity that they're experiencing in a practice. A "one" is no sensation and a "ten" is a trip to the emergency room. She suggests that they work at the intensity level of a "three" to "five," where they are experiencing sensation without straining.[76]

A lot of yoga classes with older adults include games or other activities that encourage social interaction. It's fine to make the yoga session fun and interactive, but be careful not to infantilize your older students. Always treat your students with respect and in an age-appropriate manner.

Yoga can provide support for older adults and help them to build courage as they face the challenges of aging, illness, and death. This support can be both physical, supporting the body as it ages, and emotional, offering community and comradery. Yoga can give older adults solace on a spiritual level, helping them connect with their spirit. According to Joseph Campbell:

> *The problem in middle life, when the body has reached its climax of power and begins to lose it, is to identify yourself, not with the body, which is falling away, but with the consciousness of which it is a vehicle. And when you can do that, and this is something learned from my myths, what am I? Am I the bulb that carries the light, or am I the light of which the bulb is a vehicle? And this body is a vehicle of consciousness, and if you can identify with the consciousness, you can watch this thing go, like an old car there goes the fender, there goes this. But it's expectable, you know, and then gradually the whole thing drops off and consciousness rejoins consciousness. I mean, that it's no longer in this particular environment.[77]*

Leadership

Stepping into your leadership role is very much what becoming a yoga teacher is about. Effective leaders don't just tell people what to do, they model it themselves. They also know how to guide and gather their community like a form of judo: Using the group's natural energy and power, and guiding it in the direction that they choose.

As a leader, you hold tremendous responsibility and authority, and it's important to reflect on the ways you're using that power when teaching. You need to consider how you move around the space, and the quality of your energy and presence. Are you giving equal attention to all students, or just focusing on a few?

One great thing about online teaching is that you can easily record yourself and get a sense of how you come across. For in-person classes it's harder to get a sense of yourself in this way. That's why it can be helpful to have peer support for this. You could have a yoga teacher friend who takes your classes and gives you feedback, or a group of friends who do this for each other.

Peer support means connecting with other teachers who are in a similar place in their own teaching journeys. Some people are naturally drawn to connecting with other yoga teachers, but others are more introverted and have to make a conscious effort. Not only is peer support essential for ongoing learning and feedback when you're actively teaching, but peers also provide a sounding board when you are facing a challenging situation or some issue comes up in your classes.

The other thing about being a leader is that the responsibility always lands on you. When there's disruptive behavior, or any issue in class, it's up to you to figure out how to respond. If you're teaching kids or teenagers, what is considered disruptive is different than in an adult yoga class. Similarly, if you're teaching in a non-yoga space, such as a gym, community center, or library, what is considered disruptive might be different. But in the end, you'll need to engage your practice in resolving conflict and keeping the group safe.

Personally, I have found that bringing a lightness to my teaching helps me get through those challenging times. I rely heavily on humor and humility. I'm not suggesting you make a lot of jokes, but sometimes laughter can help us bond and feel connected. Humility on your part also makes you more approachable and easier to connect with. In the end, most students don't need a perfect guru leading them, rather they need a friendly companion on their journey. I use a lot of dad jokes, but that might work for me because I'm actually a dad! One of my favorites is to ask the students to massage the sole of their foot, and then I ask them to, "Look deeply into your soul."

Scenario

You have a student, Jean, who uses a wheelchair, and she comes to class with an assistant. During class you notice that the assistant starts to move Jean's body to create the shapes that you are describing. How do you address this?

Response

This is a complicated scenario because you are dealing with an additional person, the assistant. On the one hand, the assistant can support Jean so that she can participate in class. In fact, the assistant may make it possible for her to be there by driving her and helping her get into the room. But at what point does the assistant actually interfere with Jean's experience of yoga?

From experience, I have found that it's best to have a brief conversation with both of them before class starts to clarify what will happen. Some assistants have experience in yoga settings, but most don't. My fear is that unchecked, they may actually do more harm than good by focusing just on the external shape of the poses rather than on the internal experience, and force Jean's body into unsafe positions.

Usually what I suggest is that the assistant partic-pate in the class as a student so that they can have a break and get to do some yoga. Then I'll work directly with Jeanne. Or, if I have an assistant present in class, they can support Jean. The other option is to give the assistant a lot of clear directions like, "Can you get Jean a bolster for this pose, and ask her if she would like to put it under her legs?"

The problem with this kind of situation is that once you start communicating with an assistant rather than directly with the student there may be issues with consent. If I'm meeting someone for the first time and they have an assistant present, I sometimes notice a tendency for the assistant to answer my questions rather than the student themselves. In this situation, the assistant can act as a translator, or simply step aside, so you can communicate directly with the student.

Further Reflection

• What steps can you take to make your classes more accessible? Is it the content or structure of the class that could shift?

• Have you found a balance of class preparation and spontaneity that works for you?

• What is your personal learning style or combination of styles?

• Do you have peer support? If not, how can you get it?

CHAPTER EIGHT

MAKING ASANA ACCESSIBLE

I think of adapting asana as reverse engineering a pose. I look at the ingredients of the pose and consider what gifts those different actions or ingredients are giving. This is a fun way for yoga teachers to work on sequencing. You can then explore all the ingredients of the pose in a class. You could look at all of those ingredients in different poses as well, and then put it all together. Then by the end of class, the students have a felt-sense of all the different actions, which can then be combined into some sort of final pose.

Safety, alignment, structural organization, or whatever you call it, opens up doorways to feel our body, to bring the mind's consciousness into embodiment in a different way. To feel what we were not able to feel before. When we're working with alignment, it is about keeping the body safe and honoring the design of the body.

It also creates an opportunity for awareness—to go in and to feel and experience the body in a way that you haven't before, which is huge if we're interested in re-patterning and shifting out of our old patterns of reaction in the nervous system and the mind. That's where asana relates to something like freedom or liberation because we're actually changing the way consciousness is interacting with prakriti *(nature/creation) or with our embodied reality.*

It's actually pretty vulnerable and confrontational to go in and be in your body and start to open up things that have been very guarded. To start to feel things that you have been, maybe for a good reason, trying not to feel. But if you understand the why—that there is ease and freedom and transformation, actually tangibly available—that can provide courage. As a teacher, I invite my students to have the courage to go in and feel what they have not felt before and to face the unknown.

Mostly, we have to remember that we're doing asana with the body, but it's not for the body. The body is this incredible gateway through which we can affect our mind, our emotions, our energy levels, our prana, and eventually, maybe even access a tangible experience of the soul.

—Avery Kalapa

AFTER TEACHING THOUSANDS of hours of yoga over the course of almost thirty years, many of the classes I've taught have faded from memory. But there are a number of experiences that always stay with me. One time, I was hired by the city of San Francisco to teach at a residential hospital. I didn't know who would be joining the class, and when I got there I was surprised to find five students who were all quadriplegic—meaning their bodies were mostly paralyzed. I had worked with many students with paralysis prior to that, but having five students who had almost no physical movement in a group class worried me because I wasn't sure how I could teach them.

Some of the students didn't use words to speak, so we had to explore other kinds of communication like nodding and blinking their eyes to answer yes and no questions. The attendants from the hospital had brought the students into a small conference room and left us alone, so I wasn't given much support. Needless to say, I left that first session in a slight panic that I had taken on more than I could handle.

I decided to reach out to some of my yoga teacher friends, and asked if they would be willing to assist me. Luckily two of them agreed, so we met to discuss the practices we could share in the class. It slowly dawned on me, with the inspiration of my friends, that these students were challenging me to teach yoga in a much deeper way than I was used to. I couldn't simply depend on asana the way that I was accustomed. I needed to really think about how to teach the other limbs of yoga.

By the next class, I was more prepared, and I had the support of two amazing yoga teachers. We had a variety of practices for them, and it was much more successful. The practices included gentle pranayama, imagery, meditation, and we came up with clearer ways for all the students to communicate with us and each other. After a few months, I turned that class over to one of the teachers who was assisting me, Jai Bezaire, and he ended up teaching in that facility for over a decade. The experience left me with tremendous gratitude for those students and a lot of insight about teaching yoga.

I realized that if the physical body can't, or doesn't want to, do asana you can work on a subtler layer, or kosha. The panchamaya kosha is a model of our human embodiment that describes five layers or sheaths that intertwine and intersect with each other. The five layers are the physical body, breath/energy body, mental body, intuitive body, and the bliss body.

Panchamaya Kosha—The Five Bodies

1. Annamaya kosha—physical body
2. Pranamaya kosha—energy body
3. Manomaya kosha—mental body

4. Vijnanamaya kosha—intuitive body
5. Anandamaya kosha—bliss body

If a practice isn't accessible for the physical body, you can practice on a subtler layer. You can focus on how the breath moves, or imagine the practice with the mind. This understanding had a profound shift in the way I taught all my students. I always knew that yoga was about working with the body to connect with the breath and with *prana*, life force. I also knew that it was eventually about finding peace in the mind. But the kosha model showed me how to put that into practice, and create a more accessible way in for my students. Sometimes going deeper can actually make the practice easier to grasp.

Teaching Accessible Asana

If you stop to think about it, what is it that you're actually doing when you're teaching yoga? Are you standing at the front of a room making shapes with your body and asking the students to copy you like a game of Simon Says? Or are you trying to cultivate a deeper experience? The way we cultivate that deeper experience of yoga is by working with the mind.

Yes, the body can make shapes, and we can breathe into those movements. But what makes yoga profound and transformative is what's happening in the mind. In many ways, asana is simply moving meditation. And just like with any meditative practice, the benefits come from deepening our awareness and concentration.

The result of engaging the mind in this way is magical, and yoga really is a kind of alchemy. You mix together the perfect balance of movement, breath, and focus, and poof!—the transformation occurs. You transform from feeling weighed down and worried to feeling so light you can touch the stars. Of course, each of us has our own personal alchemical recipe based on our preferences, personality, and experiences. As a yoga teacher, you're giving people guidance to create their own personal magic potion.

It's helpful to remember that asana is accessible by nature. Moving the body as a devotional practice is one of the simplest and most direct ways to practice spirituality. But somehow, in modern yoga, we've made asana exclusive, complicated, and even dangerous. There is a tradition of asceticism in yoga where the body is basically tortured as a way to transcend it—as a way of stopping the identification with the body. Contemporary asana practice seems to align itself with this part of the tradition, but there are so many other ways to practice.

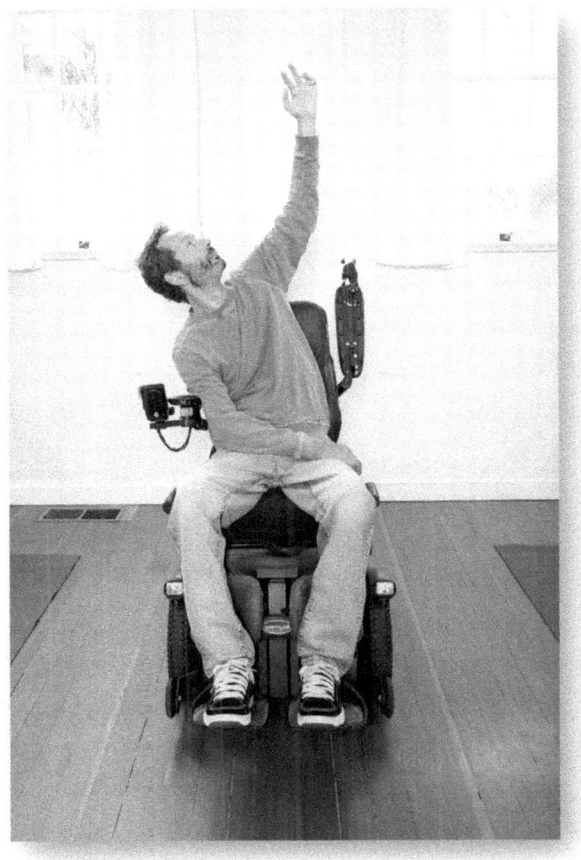

Seated side bend, parsva sukhasana

The traditional paths of yoga, which I discussed on page 61, offer a way in for all of us. There's the path of love and devotion, bhakti yoga. The path of action and service, karma yoga. The path of wisdom and self-analysis, jnana yoga, and there's the path of concentration and ethics, raja yoga.

Asana is a great support to any and all of these paths. Twisting and contorting the body by itself is not spiritual practice. But, moving the body with love is a bhakti yoga practice. Serving the body through self-care is a karma yoga practice. Reflecting on our relationship with the body as we move in and out of poses is a jnana yoga practice. Aligning breath and movement to help focus the mind is a Raja Yoga practice.

A Spectrum of Possibility

One central concept that informs all my teaching is the understanding that each yoga practice exists on a spectrum of possibility. This is similar to the concept of asana progressions, where you add elements of a practice to experience some kind of "full expression" of the pose. But this idea of a spectrum is more neutral. There are infinite ways of expressing each asana and each one is equal to the others. I've let go of the idea of "beginner" and "advanced" since they create a false dichotomy.

The idea of exploring an asana on a spectrum is more inviting and more inclusive. We can each find our special place on that spectrum of practice that is valid and effective, based on how our body, breath, and mind are experiencing this present moment.

Let's look at cobra pose, bhujangasana, as an example. This pose is essentially a backbend (spinal extension) that offers an opportunity to counteract slouching and kyphosis (rounded upper back) that happens naturally as we age. Here are twenty variations on the spectrum of possibility:

Prone:

1. A sphynx variation where you slide the hands forward and rest the forearms on the floor.
2. Place a folded blanket under the pelvis to reduce the lumbar curve.
3. Lift the hands off the floor to engage the back muscles rather than pushing with the arms.
4. Come up into the pose but lower the head to bring awareness to the thoracic spine without engaging the cervical spine.
5. Make it dynamic by coming up on the inhalation and lowering down on the exhalation.
6. Explore different leg positions; having them close together or separated, toes curled under or pointed, or squeezing a block between the legs.
7. Place a block on its highest setting under the forehead to keep the neck neutral.
8. Lie on top of a bolster so it's supporting the torso. Notice the effect on the lower back and neck.

Supine:

9. Place a bolster or folded blanket behind the upper back to create the spinal extension of cobra. Be sure to support the neck as well. This can also be done in bed.

Kneeling:

10. Lean forward and rest the hands on the knees as you come into the pose.

Standing:

11. Bend the knees slightly and rest the hands on the knees as you come into the pose.
12. Face a wall about a foot away. Bring the hands to the wall at shoulder height and come up on to the toes as you extend the spine.

Seated:

13. Place the hands on the knees and lean forward as you come into the pose.
14. In a similar position, try a dynamic movement. Exhale and lower the head down, leaning forward as if you're diving. Then as you inhale, slowly roll up the head, neck, and chest into cobra. Repeat a few times.
15. Bring the hands up in front of the shoulders as if you were on a mat, and then lean forward and come into the pose, bringing the arms back slightly to expand the chest.
16. Reach back with the hands and take hold of the back of the chair or the seat of the chair, and lean forward as you come into the pose.
17. Place a bolster, firm pillow, or blanket on the lap, and rest the arms on it. As you move forward into the pose, allow the abdomen to press gently into the prop, and pull the arms toward you as you would on the mat.
18. Scoot all the way back in the chair. Lean forward and place a folded blanket, a rolled yoga mat placed vertically, or a block behind the upper back. Lean back against the prop to find the cobra shape.
19. Seated at a desk, plant the feet and lean forward placing the hands on the edge of the desk as you come into the pose. This can also be done facing the back of a second chair or facing a wall.

Mentally:

20. Resting in shavasana, imagine practicing cobra mentally without moving. Inhabit the body and feel how it would move and how the breath would change during the practice.

[Note: In my book, *Accessible Yoga: Poses & Practices for Every Body*, I cover many specific asanas in detail with adapted versions on the chair, mat, or bed.]

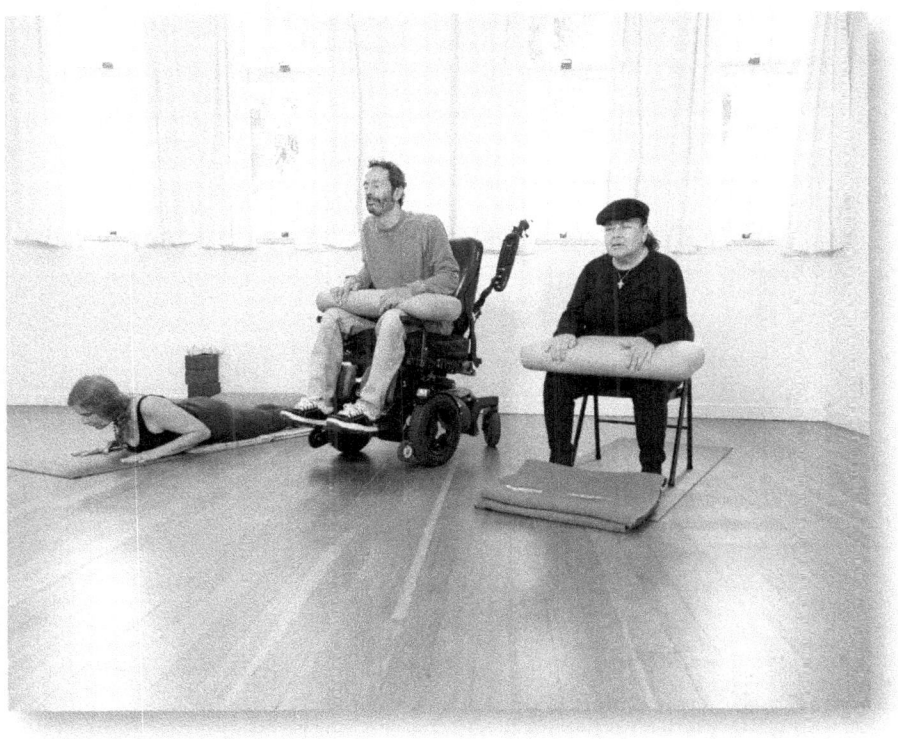

Three variations of cobra pose, bhujangasana

Find the Why

In a slightly misguided effort to be welcoming and inclusive, I've often heard yoga teachers describe poses in detail, and then as an afterthought, tell their students to "find their own version of a pose." But this feels like a bit of a cop out, even though we want everyone to make the practice their own. Beginning students in particular need clear instruction, and all students deserve equal attention and support. So, telling a student who can't do a variation of a pose that you're teaching that they should simply find their own way seems inadequate.

Without clear guidance, a student might feel like they are doing an adapted variation of a pose by trying to copy its outward appearance. But, the real challenge for teachers is to understand the purpose and structure of a pose (or group of poses) and find ways to provide the students similar benefits, working from the inside out.

Consider what experience or benefit you're trying to share with your students when teaching a particular pose. This is the most important part of adapting asana. Rather than focus just on the external appearance of a pose, think about why you practice it. Even though there may be multiple reasons for practicing a specific asana, focusing on one aspect helps make adapting more effective.

For example, if you examine vrksasana, tree pose, you find so many different components: The element of balance; strength in the supporting leg; hip opening in the raised leg; shoulder and chest opening—according to the arm position; the energetic experience of being in a tall open standing position; connecting earth and sky; and more.

To start adapting the pose, choose one element to focus on, such as balance. Then begin to reflect on how you can give everyone in the class an experience of balance in this practice. You can use this one concept to help lead you to finding creative ways to make it work for all your students. You can find ways to explore balance in supported standing versions, in the chair, or even in bed.

Doing this might call for bringing in a new element, or challenging balance in some way. In fact, my favorite chair version of tree pose is sitting tall with one leg out to the side and the heel of that foot raised onto the front leg of the chair. Then, take a foam block or eye pillow and balance it on your head. Try it, and see how it feels to bring the element of balance into a chair version of a standing balancing pose.

When thinking about the "why," you may also want to consider the "why not." Considering contraindications as well as benefits can guide you to create a safe practice. If I'm thinking of teaching downward facing dog, I also reflect on how it's a powerful inversion and would be contraindicated for people with glaucoma or high blood pressure. In that case, the challenge is to find a version of downward dog that takes away the inversion, such as practicing standing at the wall, or in a chair.

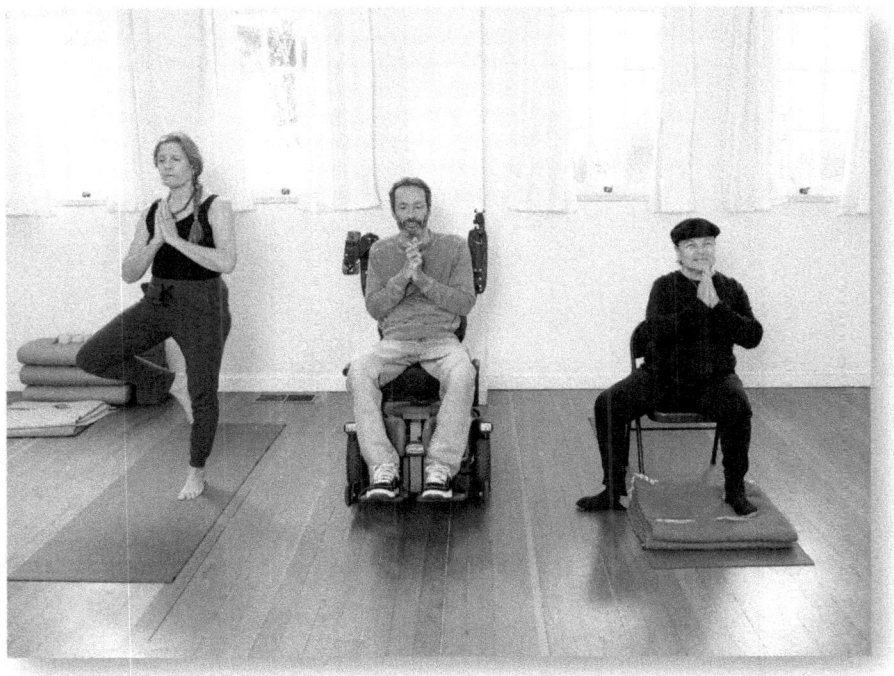

In this photo, all three students are practicing different variations of tree pose, vrksasana. *They all have their hands together at the chest, with different leg variations.*

Dissect the Pose

As I mentioned, it's helpful to begin by considering the benefits of the pose, and explore why we practice it the way we do. Then you can look at breaking it down into elements and teaching your students the portions of the pose that are accessible to them. This is similar to Avery Kalapa's concept of reverse engineering a pose, which they explained in the introduction to this chapter.

You can also remove the elements that are inaccessible. So, still using the example of downward facing dog, a student practicing a

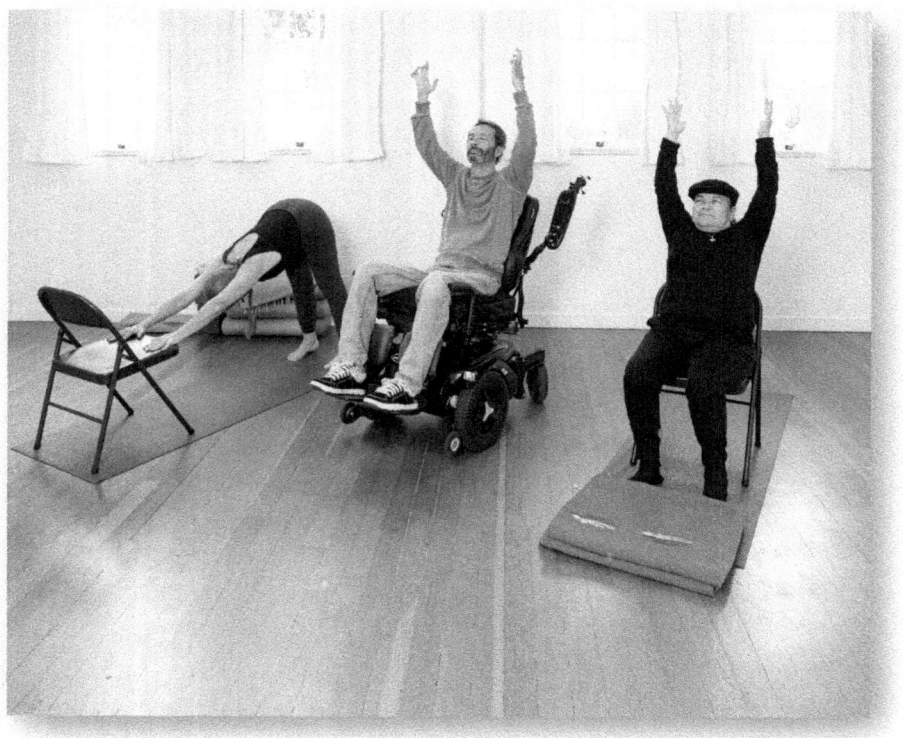

Here the students are doing three variations of downward facing dog, adho mukha svanasana. *The student on the mat has their hands on a chair to avoid a deep inversion. The other two students practicing in chairs are focused on the upper body movement.*

chair variation could potentially get the upper body action of the pose by raising the arms alongside the ears. From there, you can lead the student inward to explore lifting and lengthening the spine. This is the inner energetic experience that is essential to experiencing asana. By removing the lower body portion, which demands leg strength and balance, you can make the pose much more accessible.

Use Props

Props are a yoga teacher's best friend because they provide us ways of adapting the space around the student to fit their individual body. Props can fill space, raise the floor, connect parts of the body, add or relieve pressure, give support for balance, build structure in the pose, and much more. For example, a blanket under the hips when sitting cross-legged, such as in *sukhasana*, easy pose, can raise the floor and tilt the top of the pelvis forward making sitting more comfortable.

Props can also change the relationship between parts of the body. A strap around the extended foot in a seated forward bend, like *janushirshasana*, can help a student relax into the pose and avoid straining their lower back. In this example, the strap is also creating an energetic structure for the pose. Rather than reaching out into space with the hands, holding a strap that is connected to the foot, can give a grounded feeling that allows the body to release and let go. The strap can also help the student feel like they are connected to their foot, and help them to resist the urge to strain to touch their toes. In that way, the prop is making the pose safer.

Yoga props don't necessarily make practice easier, in fact they're completely neutral. There was even some very surprising research that showed that using yoga props may actually increase injury.[73] This might be because props can often deepen our experience of a pose.

At the same time, a small change, or the use of a simple prop, can transform someone's experience of a practice and make it accessible

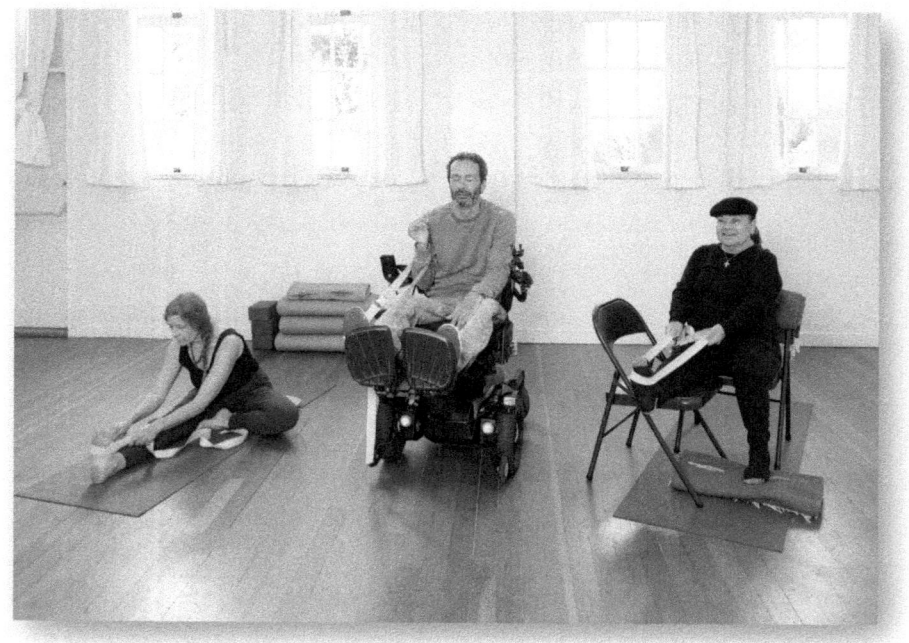

The students are doing different variations of head-to-knee pose,
janushirshasana. *All are using straps with different arm positions.*

to them. I can think of countless examples of times when I was teaching and my students needed a creative solution. Working collaboratively, we explored different options until we found a useful solution.

I remember one young woman with rheumatoid arthritis who told me she couldn't do yoga because she couldn't put weight on her hands. She was the partner of one of my students at a retreat, and told me she planned to just find other things to occupy her time while her partner came to yoga class. I asked her to come to class with the promise that if we worked together I was sure we could find a way for her to practice. So, with a little effort, we created a hands-free practice, and she was thrilled.

I remember another student who was an ex-professional dancer with extreme vertigo who couldn't lie down or even look down without getting dizzy. She had to give up dancing and all movement practices because of her condition, and it put her in a deep depression. So, working together, we created an all standing and seated practice that gave her a way back into movement and yoga.

How to Use Props

Bolsters

Bolsters are one of the more expensive yoga props, so not everyone has access to them. If a student doesn't have a bolster, and they're practicing at home, they could substitute a couch cushion, or a very firm pillow. Another option is to fold a bed pillow in half lengthwise and wrap it with a strap or towel.

Bolsters offer sturdy yet soft support for any part of the body, but are often used to support the back in backward bends, such as a supported fish pose, *matsyasana*. Or you can use a bolster to support the back of the sacrum in supported bridge pose, or low shoulderstand. A low shoulderstand is done by coming into a supported bridge. From here, take hold of the bolster with both hands, then lift the feet up and bend the knees into the chest. If that's comfortable, you can lift the legs up toward the ceiling.

Blankets

Blankets may be the most versatile of yoga props because they can quickly be folded to different heights and lengths. They can also be rolled to create the shape of a bolster or cushion. When using blankets, make sure to fold them smoothly so that the part under the body provides even support. Also, keep the smooth edge of a folded blanket toward the body, rather than the uneven side in order to have more consistent support.

Blankets can be used to add gentle weight, which can be soothing to the nervous system, as well as for warmth and a sense of protection. One of my favorite ways to use a blanket is to support the legs in sukhasana, easy pose, on the mat. Students can take a folded blanket and roll it into a shorter cylindrical shape. Then place the rolled blanket between both knees and shins. It helps lift the hips slightly, and protects the ankles, which makes sitting cross-legged for a longer period more comfortable.

Students can even roll a blanket into a long thin shape and wrap it around the back of their necks to create a support for the head in

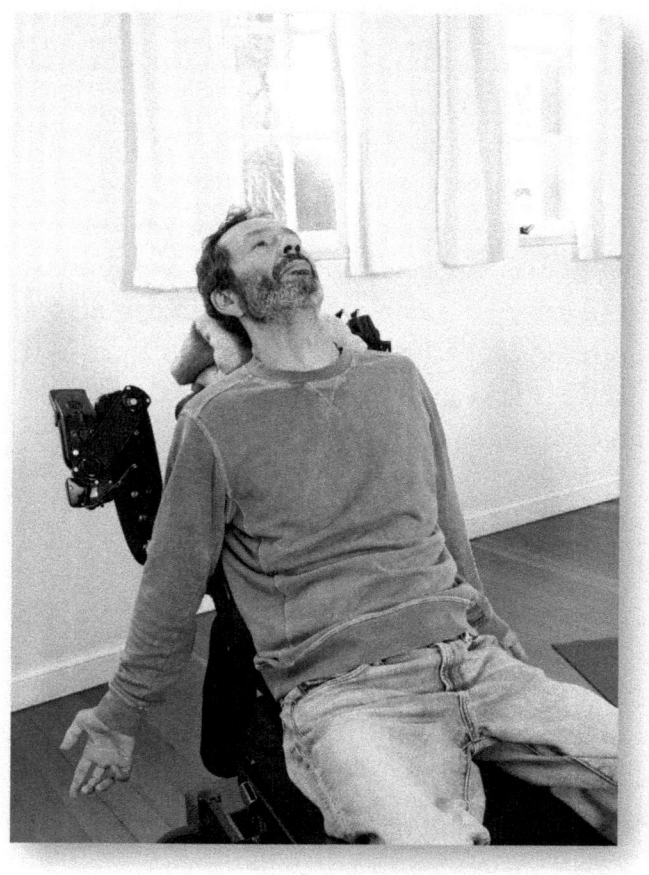

Chair matsyasana, *fish pose, with blanket support*

chair shavasana, which you can see in the photo on page 213. Generally, soft but firm blankets are best, and it's important to remember to wash them if they are being used by multiple students and classes.

Note: In many of the images in this book, the student on the right has a blanket in front of her feet. During our class, she said that because she has foot drop,[79] the weight of the blanket provided needed support. A sand bag would have also worked well for this. You can also see a way to use a blanket in the variation of fish pose in this image.

Blocks

Yoga blocks are useful when you need more firm support that won't give in to the weight of the body the way that a bolster or blanket might. Blocks can be used in standing poses, like tree, to raise the floor, or in downward dog to slightly raise the upper body. Similarly, they can support backward bends or seated poses. They can be used to create structure in the lower body by squeezing a block together between the legs.

Also, in chair yoga, blocks can provide creative solutions to strengthening practices, such as squeezing a block between the palms or the legs. Blocks can add an element of balance in chair yoga. You can balance them in the hands or on the head. Foam blocks are lightweight and relatively inexpensive, but they may not be sturdy enough for students with larger bodies. Cork or wood blocks offer much more support, but are heavier and more expensive.

Straps

Yoga straps are definitely the oldest yoga prop that we know of, and they are still being used today! (I discussed the interesting research on the history of yoga straps in chapter one.) Straps can connect parts of the body both energetically and physically as discussed above. They can create structure for the body. For example, in legs up the wall, they can help hold the legs together. They can also create or release tension by giving us something to pull on or press into.

They're useful in creating arm variations in poses like eagle and cow face pose, *gomukhasana*. In those poses, they offer something to hold onto rather than having to reach the hands together. For example, in cow face pose, you can hold the strap in the right hand and raise the right arm overhead, bending the right elbow. Then reach behind you with the left hand and take hold of the strap, walk the hands closer together until you find the right amount of stretch.

Straps are useful for connecting parts of the body without the use of the hands. For example, in a seated forward bend like janu-shirshasana, you can make a large loop with a strap and place it around the lower back and around one foot. Or, you can place the loop around the foot and in the crook of the elbows, rather than holding with the hands. This is helpful if someone has arthritis in their hands, or other conditions where they can't, or don't want to, hold a strap.

Remember, binding people with straps is not trauma-sensitive, so be cautious about the way you use them and, as much as possible, allow the students to place them on their bodies themselves.

Chairs

Obviously, chairs are an essential prop in yoga, and I think every yoga class should have them available. I already discussed chair yoga on page 126, but it's interesting to consider chairs as a general prop. Not only are chairs useful for sitting, they also provide a raised platform which can be useful in other ways. For example, in standing poses such as *trikonasana*, triangle pose, you can bring your hand down to the seat of a chair rather than trying to reach the floor. Also, the back of a chair can be useful in standing poses to help with balance.

In chair yoga, it can be helpful to have a second chair available. You can rest forward on it in a chair child's pose, or rest the feet on it for many different kinds of forward bends. You can also use a second chair to raise the legs and offer a gentle inversion. In fact, for mat practice, instead of having students practice legs up the wall pose, they can rest their lower legs on the seat of a chair for a slightly less intense inversion.

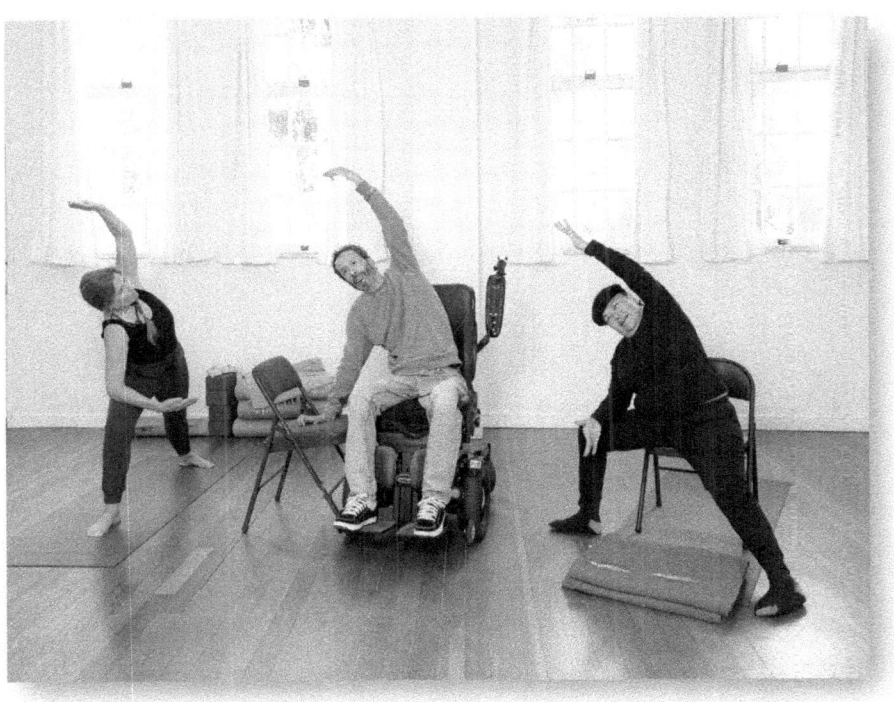

Three students practicing extended side angle pose, utthita parsvakonasana. *In the middle, one student is bringing their hand to the seat of a chair rather than to their leg.*

Walls

Walls are the most underrated yoga prop. They can give support to a student doing standing poses, either by having their back against the wall, or reaching toward the wall with a hand. A wall can be used in chair yoga in poses like downward dog, or *chaturanga,* four-limbed staff pose, or other places where you're reaching out with the arms by sitting facing a wall.

The wall can be used in mat practice to support the feet and create a sense of grounding if you're practicing standing poses in a reclined format. For example, you can practice a reclined tree pose with the foot of your supporting leg pressing into a wall, and feeling the pressure grounding you as if it was the floor. In mat downward dog, students with tight hamstrings or those needing extra support can practice with the heels against the wall. That variation can make the pose much more accessible. You can also lean against the wall in seated poses, and use the wall for supported inversions like legs up the wall.

Mats

If you've ever practiced yoga in the sand or on grass you know that floors are also an important yoga prop, as are yoga mats. We often take them both for granted, but hard floors and mats provide resistance which is an important element to consider in asana practice. Rolled mats can also be used like small, thin bolsters. They can be rolled loosely and placed behind a student's back in a chair to help with mountain pose, *tadasana.* Or they can be used under the front of the ankles in child's pose, *balasana.*

Keep in mind that the resistance of a mat can be too much in certain circumstances. For example, if students choose to wear their shoes in class, their shoes might stick to the mat as they walk around, and create a tripping hazard. I'll also mention that it's important to be open to people wearing their shoes in yoga class for a variety of reasons. They may have trouble taking them on and off, or their shoes might have special orthotics or braces. Often these supports make students feel more stable with their shoes on, and that's important. So demanding that people remove their shoes is not necessary.

Similarly, if people have prosthetic limbs it is completely up to them to decide whether or not to wear them in class. Prosthetics, crutches, wheelchairs, and any assistive devices or mobility aids should be considered parts of people's bodies and should never be touched or moved without consent. This also includes eyeglasses and hearing aids.

Be Creative

Creativity is an expression of spirituality, and it becomes yoga if it's offered in the light of service. If you are teaching a student who is struggling with a particular practice, consider creative ways to make them more comfortable or to adapt the practice to them, rather than the other way around. Creativity used in this way is a powerful tool of accessibility.

I remember working with one student who had a severe form of arthritis that caused her to have multiple joint replacements. One day, she was in a class where I was teaching eagle pose, and we couldn't find any way to practice that was comfortable for her. She said that practicing in a chair bothered her hips, and when she was standing she was afraid she would fall over, even if her back was against a wall. Luckily there was a thin pillar in the middle of the room, so I suggested she gently hug it with her arms. She was so excited and said that she experienced the pose in her body for the first time because she felt secure and balanced.

It was a moment of inspiration that I couldn't have planned, and may not have recommended to a different student. Knowing her particular challenges, and that she was willing to try new things, encouraged me to offer a rather unusual solution.

Reflection

Can you engage your intuition and creativity in service of your students?

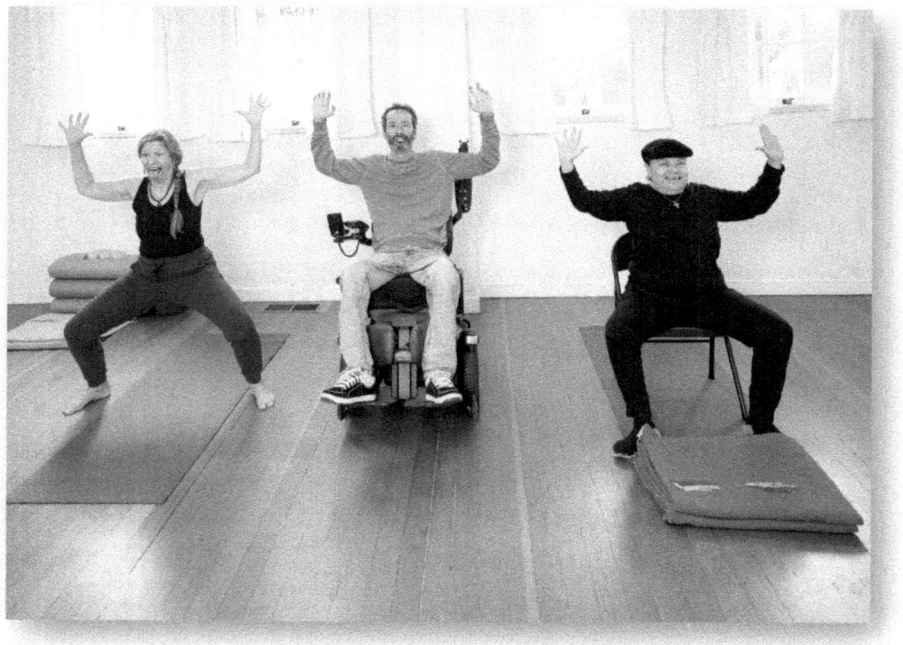

Goddess pose, utkata konasana

Collaborate

In many ways, this example of my student who practiced eagle pose with a pillar shows the benefits of student-teacher collaboration. Even though I made the suggestion, I could feel her willingness to try something new. She had a collaborative spirit, and that allowed me to be more adventurous with my solutions.

Oftentimes, students come up with the best variations of practices themselves. I know I said that we shouldn't simply tell them to "find their own version of a pose." But, with some guidance, there is a give and take that occurs between student and teacher that can lead to the most amazingly creative and inspired solutions.

I've learned so much from my students in this regard, and I think it's important to honor their choices, as long as you feel that they are practicing safely. Collaboration means that you work together to find a solution, and generally speaking, two heads are better than one when trying to solve a problem.

I had a longtime student who had some major issues with her neck, and although she liked to practice on a mat, she was never comfortable practicing prone poses like cobra. I suggested she practice in a chair, but she was resistant to doing that. So I suggested she try practicing standing. She tried that a few times, but wasn't sure about it. Then one day, she got into a kneeling position and practiced cobra from there. It was a brilliant solution because she could lean forward enough to put some weight into her hands, and get a similar spinal movement. It was easier for her to keep her neck long in that version, and she felt stable, so it provided a safer and more effective variation for her.

Change Orientation / Effects of Gravity

One thing I always consider when adapting practice is what format my students will be most comfortable in: standing, seated, lying in bed, or getting on the floor. Can they put pressure on their hands and wrists, and are there other mobility limitations to be aware of? Would practicing the same shape but in a different orientation be more accessible?

Another way to adapt an asana is to change the body's orientation in space, and therefore change the way that gravity affects the body. For example, for someone with tight hamstrings, a seated forward bend, such as *paschimottanasana*, can be challenging. If the person is sitting on the ground with their legs extended in front of them in *dandasana*, staff pose, and is unable to bring their torso perpendicular to the floor, then they are working against gravity to lift and lengthen their spine. The pose becomes a sit up in that position. To begin moving forward into paschimottanasana from there would probably be a strain on their back, especially if they have preexisting back issues.

Instead, *uttanasana*, a standing forward bend, allows the student to use gravity to move more safely into a forward bend. Or *supta padangustasana*, reclining hand to big toe pose, provides a way to practice forward bending where the spine is completely neutral and supported by the floor.

Make It Dynamic

Sometimes adding movement to asana can make it more accessible. Moving into and out of a pose with the breath, which is called dynamic practice, can be a gentler experience than holding a pose in a more static way. For example, coming into bhujangasana, cobra, on an inhalation, and coming out on an exhalation can be a useful way of exploring the practice.

At the same time, some students may struggle with integrating the breath and movement. In that case, it can be helpful to start with just focusing on movement and then integrate the breath later. Cat-cow gives a way to explore dynamic movement, and works well on a chair. Just be careful to limit the spinal flexion of cat pose for students practicing in a chair. As I mentioned on page 150, spinal flexion may not be helpful in chair yoga if the student is slouching or has kyphosis.

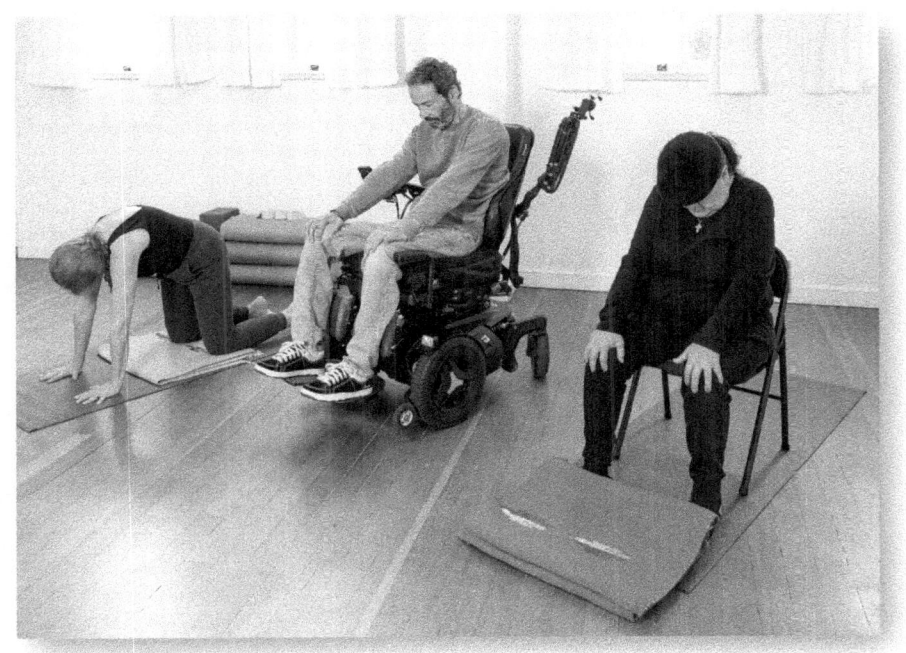

Cat pose, marjaryasana

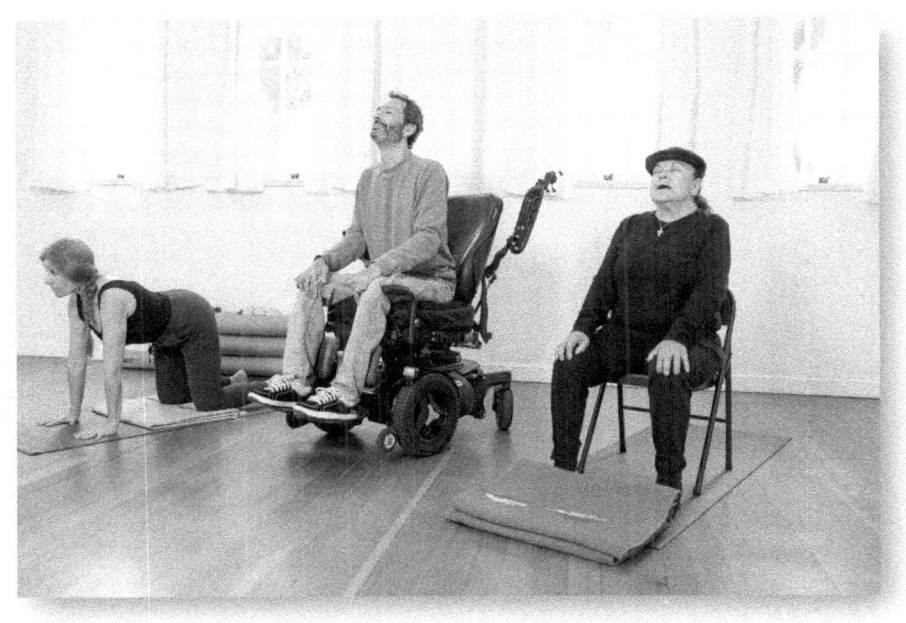

Cow pose, bitilasana

Use Inner Experience

Sometimes when we can't find a form of a pose that works for a student, we tell them to imagine the pose in their mind. On the one hand, it can feel like we're shirking our responsibility, but on the other hand, it's an opportunity to explore the inner experience of an asana. Visualizing a posture or practice is actually a very subtle and powerful way to practice. They can experience many of the benefits of a pose by imagining doing it in the mind. In fact, sports medicine has been researching the benefits of visualization for reducing athletes' performance anxiety and for helping them stay in shape when practice isn't possible.[80]

Additionally, practicing in the mind can offer an opportunity to explore the energetics of the practice. Students can feel the experience of a pose in the body even as they are imagining it. Generally, this technique works best for students who already have an asana practice and may be able to use sensory recall to recreate the feeling of being in a particular pose.

Reflection

Lie in shavasana, and without moving the body, imagine practicing one of your favorite poses, or a round of sun salutation. Rather than observing from the outside, try to feel the embodied experience of the practice, even breathing with the movements.

What's Wrong with Saying "Modification?"

It's important to be cognizant of the language we use when we teach yoga. I'm not saying we need to pause before every word, or that we'll never make mistakes. I make mistakes all the time! What I mean is that we need to become more conscious of our word choice because the spoken word is the medium of yoga teaching. Just as an artist uses colored paints, we use words to help illustrate and shape our students' experience. It's important to reflect on the reality that we are painting with our words.

For example, I don't love the terms "modification" and "modify" when it comes to discussing asana. I don't think modification is an offensive word, but I think it connects to pose hierarchy, and reflects a limited way of thinking of asana. Typically, in yoga contexts, "modification" infers that something is reduced or watered-down. In fact, one of its definitions is "limitation or qualification."[81]

Although I'm specifically talking about an English word, this may apply to other languages as well. I actually think adapting a practice for someone doesn't make it less than. Rather, you're expanding it and making it more. So I like to find words that reflect the feeling of adding on, such as, "vary/variation," or "adapt/adaptation," or even, "choose your own adventure."

To Demo or Not to Demo, That Is the Question

Demoing will make your classes more accessible for visual learners, students who are Deaf/deaf or hard of hearing, as well as those who speak a different language than you do. I've taken yoga classes in German, Spanish, Italian, and French, none of which I'm fluent in. While the use of Sanskrit names made it possible for me to participate in those classes, demos made it so much easier and meant I didn't have to stare at the other students.

When demoing, it's important to remember that students will often try to copy the teacher. I remember one time, I was teaching alternate nostril breathing and I had a new student in the front of the class. At one point, I took my hand away from my nose to scratch my head and the student copied me and scratched their head!

Students see you as the expert and they may think they are expected to perform whatever version of a pose you are doing. This can be dangerous and misleading. So, when demonstrating in class, be aware of the version of the pose that you choose to show. Generally, I recommend demonstrating the gentlest version (often in a chair) so that the students practicing at that level feel represented. Or, if you have students practicing in a chair, at least spend a portion of the class demonstrating from a chair.

Also, when demonstrating, try not to get absorbed into your personal practice. You only do what is needed to help the students understand the practice, and keep your eyes on them. Also, make sure you can still project your voice when demoing. I've been in classes where teachers are facing their mat or facing away from the students, and I can't hear what they're saying.

One of the worst experiences I ever had in yoga was when I took the class of a well-loved yoga teacher in a very large room. It was packed, and I was in the back of the room. The teacher stood on his mat speaking very quietly in his yoga voice the entire time without a mic, and I couldn't hear a word he was saying, and he wasn't demoing anything. I even asked him to speak up, and it didn't help. I ended up just copying the practice of the students around me, and it was incredibly frustrating. It reminded me how important it is that all the students can hear us or see us at all times.

Teaching Integrated Classes

As yoga teachers, we need to help our students find safe and effective ways to practice, whether online or in person. One of the most helpful ways of doing this is to give a few variations and options for every practice that we teach. In this way, you can create integrated classes where students are practicing at multiple levels at the same time and no one is made to feel less than the others.

As much as possible, you can avoid some students feeling like they're doing the "real" practice while the others are working toward that. Instead, there is a focus on unity and connection among the entire class. All the students can focus on the subtle aspects, such as interoception, breath, energy, and mind, rather than struggle with feelings of inadequacy.

An integrated class may mean that some students are practicing on the mat and some are practicing in chairs. Or, all may be using a mat or all using chairs, but there are many different variations happening at the same time.

The way I approach this is by making sure that my instruction integrates all the students into the same practice rather than teaching a version of a practice to one group of students and then separately teaching a different practice to another group, which tends to be the default method that most teachers use.

For example, they'll teach one practice like triangle pose, trikonasana, all the way through, and then notice someone struggling in the pose. Then they'll offer a variation of the practice to that one student who is struggling. Even though they mean well, when they do this it sets up a scenario where one person or group feels separate, and even less than, the others.

This problem is even more obvious when a student is practicing in a chair when the majority of the class is on the mat. What I've seen in those situations is that the student using a chair will often hide in the back of the room, and the teacher will mostly ignore them, hoping they can, "find their own modifications." This goes against the basis of yoga philosophy which speaks to our universal connection. Instead this scenario expresses separation and segregation based solely on ability.

The approach I'm suggesting is similar to the principle of *krama*,[32] or the step-by-step approach that is taught in some yoga traditions. With that approach, students are offered practices that lead up to a full pose, similar to a pose progression. That is an effective technique for many students, but it is based on the idea of constantly improving and achieving more and more physically challenging poses. What I'm describing here is slightly different. I'm suggesting that you offer different variations of a practice at the same time, and that you give them equal value. They don't exist only as a stepping stone to something else.

Offering instructions that include everyone in class at once is an approach that is similar to adaptive teaching,[83] which is used in primary education as a way to integrate disabled students into general classroom settings. It can take some preparation and experience, and I have a few tips that can help.

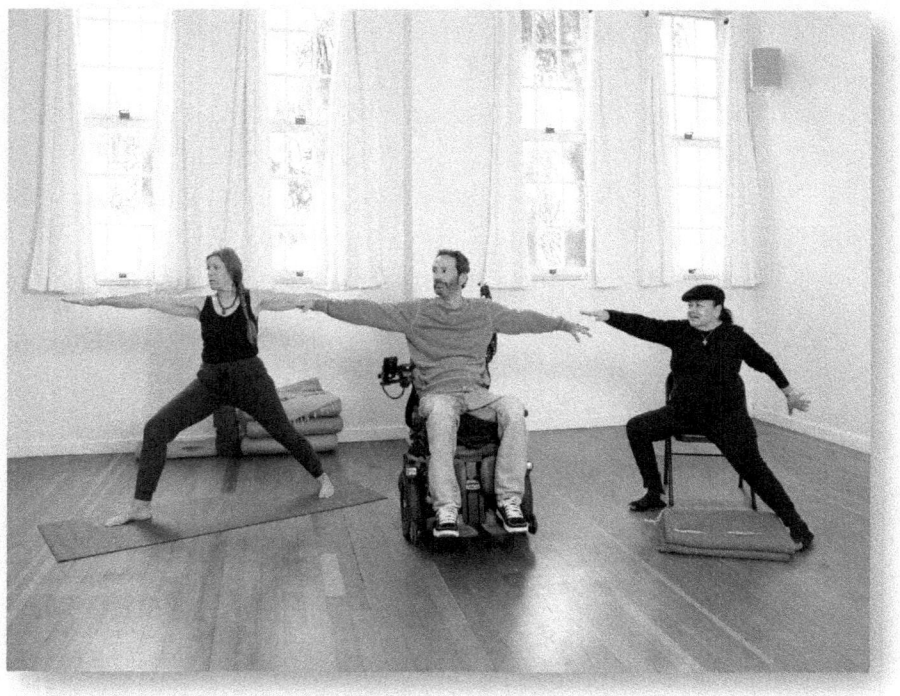

Three students practicing variations of warrior 2, virabhadrasana 2 *in an integrated classroom environment, where some are in chairs and another is standing on a mat.*

Prepare Separately, Practice Together

To cultivate a truly unified experience, I use a technique that I call *prepare separately, practice together*. The idea is to help students find the appropriate preparatory position, or foundation of a pose, according to the orientation that they're using—mat, chair, standing, etc. These are taught separately, so that students have a safe entry point into the practice. Then, I figure out what are the shared or universal aspects of the practice that everyone can do together.

For example, if I'm teaching *ardha matsyendrasana*, half spinal twist, to a group where some students are practicing in a chair and some are on the mat, I need to prepare the chair and mat students *separately*. I might teach the preparatory position on the chair first, having those students choose to turn to the right side of their chair, sitting sideways, and cross their right leg over the left, or not.

On the mat, I would have students prepare the foundation of the pose by sitting with both legs extended out in front of them. Then bend the right knee and cross the right foot over the left leg, and hold the right knee with the left hand, or bend the right knee and bring the right foot to the floor without crossing it over the leg.

Then, in order to practice together, I would give universal instructions for everyone to come into the fullness of the pose together. So the next set of instructions might sound like this:

"Everyone, bring the left hand to the right knee, and the right hand to the chair or floor behind you. Inhale and lengthen your spine. As you exhale, slowly twist around to the right, gently looking to your right. On each inhale see if you can feel the spine lengthening and each exhale supporting a gentle twist in the middle and upper back."

After a few breaths, I'd continue, "To come out of the pose, on the next exhale slowly return to center, releasing the hands and the legs, and notice how you're feeling."

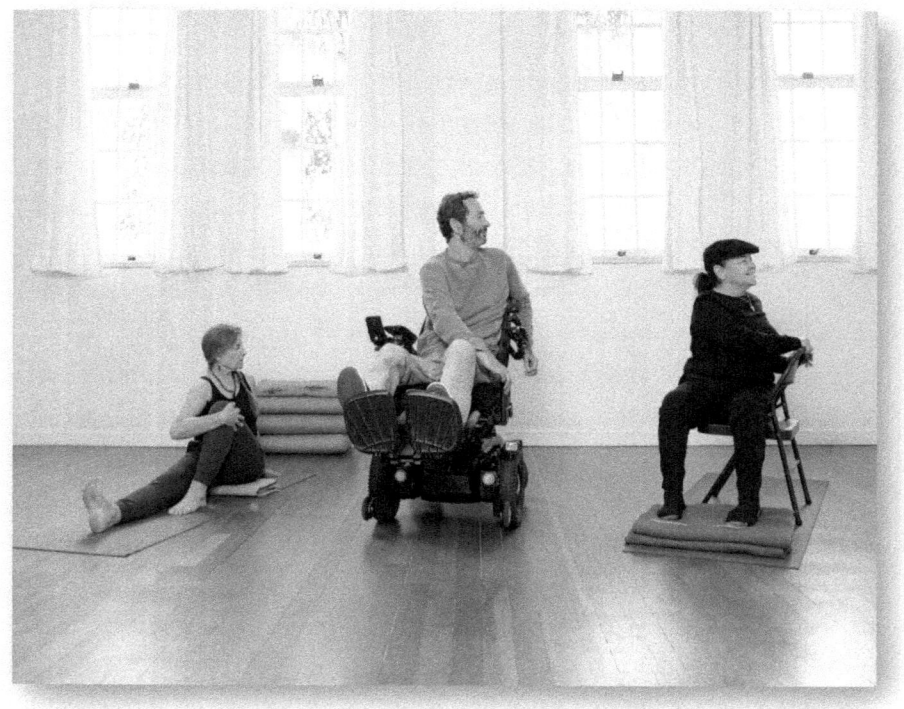

An integrated class practicing ardha matsyendrasana, *half spinal twist.*

The goal of integrated Accessible Yoga classes is to create a welcoming environment for all students, and to cultivate a feeling of inclusiveness among them. The intention here is to maximize the amount of time that students practice in unison. In addition, an integrated class requires a commitment to accommodation that is woven into thoughtful preparation. There are certain postures that lend themselves to be taught in this way. For example, eagle pose, *garudasana*, chair pose, *utkatasana*, and seated twists are some of the easiest to teach simultaneously in different orientations.

With this technique, you don't always have to begin by teaching the students in the chair. You would begin with the students who could comfortably hold the preparatory position for a longer period of time. Teaching yoga sometimes feels like simultaneously patting your head and rubbing your belly—doing two, or sometimes three, things at once, so give yourself a break if it feels overwhelming.

To summarize, here are some useful tips for teaching truly integrated classes:

- Prepare separately, practice together
- Start from the foundation and build up
- Find common movements
- If it's too complicated to teach multiple variations at the same time, at least bring the students into the pose separately and then instruct them to breathe together

Adapting Vinyasa

It can be challenging to create this same type of integrated experience in a fast or flowing asana series. But it works if you have time to prepare a flow that can be done both in a chair and on a mat. If possible, keep the lower body or foundation of the pose stable, or with minor shifts of position, and focus the movements in the spine and upper body. For example, a warrior flow can work really well this way.

To teach a mixed-level sun salutation, you need to do some preparation ahead of time. You can start by finding a chair version of each of the poses in the version of sun salute that you are teaching. Then practice in a chair yourself, and see if you can create a similar flow that matches up to the mat version. When teaching this, either start by teaching everyone the chair version and then give students the option to come to standing or to stay in a chair. Or you can experiment with demoing the chair version while you give verbal instructions for the mat series. Of course, this works best if some of your students are experienced. If you have a large class, it's also helpful to have an assistant who can demonstrate one version of the practice while you demo the other.

The wall is also an incredibly useful prop when adapting a flowing asana series. If someone wants an adapted flow and is willing to practice standing, they can use the wall for support. Students practicing in a chair can also move to face a wall. And the poses that involve reaching down to the floor (e.g., *adho mukha svanasana*, downward facing dog, plank, chaturanga) can be adapted by bringing the hands to the wall instead. With some creativity and collaboration, you can imagine the wall is like the floor and create a more accessible flow.

In vinyasa classes, teachers usually cue one breath per movement, but it doesn't need to be done that way. Experiment with two or more breaths per movement, and notice how you can slow your flow and create a more conscious and accessible flowing series in that way.

Scenario

A new student who uses a wheelchair comes to your class. You advertise the class as All Levels, but all the other students practice on the mat. What do you do?

Response

There is so much to say about this—I guess that's why I wrote a whole book about it! But the first thing I would say is to not make any assumptions about someone because they use a wheelchair. Mostly, don't assume they can't walk or stand or get on the floor.

If possible, the best thing to do is to talk to new students about whether they have experience with yoga, and what orientation they are most comfortable practicing in. For example, do they want to stay in their wheelchair, transfer to a hard chair, get on a mat, etc.?

You don't need to, or even have the right to, ask them why they use a wheelchair. All you need to do is focus on how they can safely participate in the class and have the best experience possible. I discussed this in detail in chapter two, but understanding your scope of practice is essential.

If the student plans to practice in a chair, then you can make them more comfortable by demoing at least part of the class from a chair. Also, I would encourage the student not to hide in the back of the room, but to choose a space right alongside those practicing on a mat. If possible, having their body facing the same direction as the other students will make your cueing easier—especially if you're going to instruct chair and mat versions of poses in the integrated style I described earlier. Also, everyone is different, so one person might be shy and want limited attention, and another might relish your attention. So it's important to not assume that someone practicing in a wheelchair, or a chair, needs more help than the other students.

In the very first yoga class that I ever taught, I had a big group of over twenty students and at the last minute an older woman came in with her leg in a cast and using crutches. At first I assumed that she would need more help than I could provide as a brand new teacher. But the moment we started moving, I could see that she was actually an extremely experienced practitioner. That was a lesson I'll never forget—avoid stereotypes and judgments.

Sometimes, if I see someone doing something unusual in class, I notice my mind assumes they don't know what they're doing. To counteract that urge, I try to approach the student with genuine curiosity and assume they have made a conscious choice. I'll say something like, "That's an interesting choice. Can you tell me about it?"

PART THREE

TEACHING SUBTLE PRACTICES

CHAPTER NINE

TRAUMA-SENSITIVE TEACHING

It's important for yoga teachers, and all people, to understand that a lack of bodily agency is very common after experiencing trauma. For teachers, the most important thing we can do is create an environment and offer tools that can help bring back that sense of agency—to create a very choice-oriented space so that people have the agency to choose to do something, or to not do something, in your class.

Trauma is often experienced as something that's moving, living, breathing, expanding, and contracting in the body. So as a teacher or guide, you need to be awake to the small subtle cues that you are sending your students, like for example, making eye contact with some students but not others. We must be aware of the subtle messages that we're sending our students because they will likely pick up on them.

It's also important that we, as guides, embody a regulated nervous system and that our presence makes clear that we have an open, compassionate heart toward all—that we're really listening and seeing people from our hearts. That creates safety. It allows for co-regulation for folks who are not yet ready to really connect deeply with their own bodies, or maybe can connect for a moment, but then must disconnect because their nervous systems aren't ready for that.

For those folks, self-regulation is challenging, and the beauty of yoga is that it helps to build self-regulation, which is a skill that's established over time. That's where the importance of co-regulation comes in. Co-regulation means that as the guide, if our nervous system is regulated, we can then help other nervous systems regulate simply because those nervous systems are in the presence of our nervous system. This means we have to be doing our own work as yoga teachers so that we can remain regulated and able to tolerate some level of distress should it arise in order to support the other people in the room.

It's so important that we continue to do our own work. Because when we are in the role of teacher, we are in a seat of power. And with that seat of power, there's the power to help and the power to harm. We all have the capacity to do harm, either intentionally or unintentionally. So we must continually ask ourselves how we can continue to work on ourselves and explore, because that's what yoga is about, right? That's the practice of svadhyaya *(self study).*

— Nityda Gessel

YOU CAN'T MAKE yoga accessible without being trauma-sensitive. But, both terms get tossed around so much these days that I'm afraid they may lose their meaning. To me, trauma-sensitive teaching means respecting each student's autonomy and agency, and giving them control over their own practice. As I discussed in detail in chapter five, agency and consent are the key elements that make a practice both accessible and trauma-sensitive. Agency is cultivated through your approach and attitude when teaching more than it is through the specific words you use or practices that you lead or adapt.

The first step is to reflect on your role and consider what it is you're trying to accomplish. Are you trying to fix or heal your students, or can you perceive them as already full and complete? This is a very different perspective than seeing students as traumatized and needing to be healed. And it may change the way you view your role as teacher. In fact, "teacher" may start to feel like the wrong term for sharing tools that connect people back to themselves. Maybe "guide" is better, or "companion along the path."

Humanity & Spirituality

Over the years, I've had many students talk about finding healing in my classes. Some talked about feeling safe in a group for the first time in their lives. Some talked about how yoga gave them insight into their own personal story, and how that insight offered new perspectives and a shift in the way they felt about their past. At the same time, I've had people walk out of my classes and never return. I realize that each of us has a completely unique history and related trauma, and what works for one of us won't work for the others. I can only do my best and leave the rest.

I know that when I affirm my students' fundamental humanity I am encouraging them to embrace all of themselves, especially their differences. These differences include their diverse lived experiences and past traumas, and it includes the sizes and shapes of their bodies, their ethnicities, genders, sexualities, mental health statuses, and disabilities. All of these differences make up the kaleidoscopic beauty of each person's individuality and reflect the beauty of their essential nature. That's the paradox of yoga's fundamental teaching: We're all different and special, but deep in our hearts, we're the same.

My experience is that when we feel outcast, discarded, or excluded, we can tap into an inner strength that can guide us. Sometimes it leads us to yoga. There is a famous Latin saying, *"Ad astra per aspera,"* which means, "To the stars through difficulty," which I feel expresses the heart of what we're doing when we're teaching yoga. We're not asking our students to deny their suffering and challenges with spiritual bypassing in order to connect with some ethereal inner peace. Instead, we're asking them to integrate their humanity with their spirituality by completely embracing the sharp, painful parts of themselves that hurt to touch.

We're not discarding our humanity to be "spiritual." To be guided by humanity is to allow the diversity of our lives to blossom into something really powerful—a new way of being in the world and of being with each other that can free us all.

Personally, I thought I had processed most of my major issues which arose from being a closeted queer kid, and then surviving the AIDS crisis. Yoga provided me tremendous healing, but there is always more to do. Then, a few years ago, when my mother died, something was triggered in me. I had a major panic attack that landed me in the emergency room.

I feel like I'm finally stable again, but after her death it took me years to process the trauma that I was reliving and my nervous system's response. It was like starting over with my yoga practice, which I found very frustrating. But in the end, I feel grateful for the opportunity to be a beginner again, and to notice which parts of my practice feel soothing, and which ones aren't. Once again, my practice is a cool breeze calming the prickly heat of my anxiety, and I feel such gratitude for the teachings and for all my teachers. And even more than before, I feel the need to share these teachings with anyone else who is similarly overwhelmed, stressed, and anxious.

The Teacher-Student Relationship

The first step in making your teaching trauma-informed is to identify the power dynamics within the teaching space. With awareness of these dynamics, there is an opportunity to address them consciously, and to find ways to balance them out. The teacher-student relationship is by definition imbalanced. The teacher has power and authority that the student doesn't. But you have an opportunity to address that, and even change it, in the way you run your classes. I discussed this in the earlier chapter on power and consent, but because it's so important, I'd like to revisit it here.

Consider whether the students are given a voice, and how receptive you are to hearing it. Ask yourself if there are nonverbal cues that reinforce your authority, and work to remove those. Those might include the way you move around the space, or the spoken and unspoken rules you apply. For example, can students leave early without criticism? Can they skip a practice if they feel like it? Are they allowed to speak during class?

Reflection

How would it make you feel if a student ignored your instruction and did a practice that was authentically theirs?

I remember when I was just starting to teach and someone would come to class and completely do their own practice, ignoring my instruction. I would get so frustrated and confused, although I usually just left them alone. It took a few years for me to realize that, once again, I was making it personal. I thought their behavior was a reflection on my teaching. In fact, it was simply their practice, and I was allowing them to have the space for it. These days, if I see a student doing that I'm thrilled (as long as they're not doing anything that's dangerous for them or anyone else).

It's also taken me many years to realize that asking students to sense what's happening in their bodies or with their breath might actually be triggering. And it took my own experience with anxiety to really understand it. So, I've learned patience, and that it can take time to bring awareness within. Always offer students the option of not doing a practice or doing a different variation that feels safer for them.

Often trauma-sensitive yoga is summarized by the idea of using invitational language when teaching, but that may not always work. Invitational language means that rather than speaking in commands you speak with invitations, such as, "If it feels good, try bringing your arm up." In theory, it's a wonderful way to teach, but I've found that for some students with trauma, and with new students in general, it's a lot to ask.

Trauma can make it difficult, if not impossible, for people to sense how they're feeling. So, they often need to take the process of noticing how they feel slowly and build that muscle. I try to find a balance between inviting students to explore how they feel, and giving very straight-forward, clear instructions that are easy to follow. I give a general invitation toward the beginning of class to make the practice their own, and remind them of that goal occasionally. I'll say things like, "Remember, this is your practice, so feel free to adapt or stop if something is uncomfortable."

As with everything in life, there is a middle path. That is also true of the content of your classes—the practices you teach and the props you use. While straps can be a useful prop for making many poses more accessible, some students may be disturbed by the sense of restriction that straps, or other props, can create. In fact, it's important to protect the students from the feeling of both being too restricted, and also of being too exposed. Again, it's a fine balance.

Over time, yoga practice can be beneficial in reducing the symptoms of trauma. But it's a very personal and individual journey. The best we can do as teachers is to provide a neutral and safe container for that healing to occur. That healing journey includes assisting students in learning to recognize and accept physical sensations and thereby regain a feeling of safety inside their bodies.

Here are some tips for creating a trauma-sensitive environment in all your yoga classes. If you work with populations that may have more trauma, such as in prisons or residential treatment centers, than additional specific training may be necessary:

- During centering, shavasana, pranayama, and meditation, yoga teachers usually tell people to close their eyes, but some people find discomfort in the darkness. The feeling of safety is important, so we can suggest that students who prefer not to close their eyes keep a fixed gaze on a spot while letting their focus soften and relax. Another option is to relax their gaze and be conscious of their peripheral vision. Trauma can make us extremely focused, so relaxing the gaze in this way can be a powerful practice.
- Allow students to choose where they want to position themselves in the space as long as it doesn't interfere with other students. Some people like to have their back to a wall or be able to see the door from where they are sitting.
- Avoid touching students—even hugging them before or after class. If you need to touch, make sure you have clear consent at all times. If you feel the need to walk around class and interact with students individually, you could bring people props, or adjust props for them, without touching their bodies.
- Consider each person's mat to be their private space. Don't sneak up on someone from behind, and don't enter into that space without their permission.
- Avoid letting students touch each other unless you've advertised that you're doing partner work. Students may be inappropriate with each other or may injure each other by accident.
- In online classes, offering the option to have videos off may help students feel safer.

- Having emergency contact information for all your students is essential, whether you are teaching in person or online. Also, first aid and CPR training is essential if you're teaching in-person classes.

- If a student is threatening harm to themselves or others it is appropriate to reach out for support for them. This could mean asking if they have someone you can call for them. If it's an emergency situation, it means calling the appropriate emergency services. Also, don't hesitate to get help if you feel overwhelmed or unsafe.

- Avoid sexual innuendo or positions that may make students feel exposed or unsafe. In fact, encourage practices and poses that feel protected and safe. For example, covering the body in shavasana even if it's not cold, but to provide the weight and the protection of a blanket. If it's very warm, the students can place a folded blanket just over their abdomen or anywhere that feels comfortable.

- Keep the lights on during class. Dimming them during shavasana is okay if it's still bright enough to easily see. If students prefer darkness in shavasana they can bring an eye pillow to class, or use a sleeve of a shirt to cover their eyes.

- Don't let other people observe your class, whether it's other yoga teachers or an interested student. It would be better for someone to participate rather than sit staring at the other students.

- Don't photograph your students or record your online classes without explicit permission. If you need publicity photos, plan a photoshoot that is specifically for that purpose.

- Protect your students' privacy as much as possible. This means keeping their personal information confidential as well as any other information they share with you. Also, encourage students' to protect each other's privacy. If you have any sharing time in class, students should understand that those personal stories are also private.

- If you use music, try to use neutral music that's unlikely to trigger memories or specific emotional responses.
- Avoid using scented candles, incense, or essential oils. Smells can trigger memories, not to mention that students may be allergic or have chemical sensitivity.
- Try to teach in a physical space that has minimum interruptions such as other people coming in and out.
- During shavasana and meditation, or any time you're encouraging students to close their eyes, try to avoid walking around the room or letting other students walk around. In those quiet, inward moments it can be particularly helpful to do whatever you can to create a sense of safety.

The Impact of Trauma

Trauma-informed teaching means that we assume that all our students have had some kind of trauma in their lives, and that we teach in a way that provides a space for healing from trauma, rather than triggering it. There are many different kinds of trauma including acute trauma from a single incident, chronic trauma from prolonged ongoing exposure, or complex trauma from multiple traumatic events. There is also race and ethnic based trauma,[84] and the trauma that members of all marginalized communities face on a daily basis.

There is also amazing research on the impact trauma has on multiple generations of families. Trauma doesn't necessarily change our genetic structure, but it can change the ways that our genes express themselves. This can have an impact on mental and physical health for generations. But it also means that we have an opportunity to heal ourselves and our descendants.[85]

This is what it means to be a living ancestor, and to reflect on our location in the stream of humanity, past and future. We can heal the past and we can heal the future by healing ourselves. In her book, *We*

Heal Together, Michelle Cassandra Johnson shares a practice about recognizing our place in the unbroken lineage that we have inherited:

> *You embody all the stories, narratives, experiences, and memories of your ancestors. Notice your patterns and the people and the things you are drawn to. Notice the music you love to listen to and the foods you enjoy eating. Notice how you move in your body, what blocks there are to your movements, and where ease exists within your body. Notice your voice and hear the resonance of your ancestors in it. Notice your aversions and the things you love.*
>
> *Since you are made manifest because of your ancestors, the entirety of who you are and how you show up in the world is a map for understanding more about where you come from. Observe and record your observations even if you cannot explain where certain traits you embody come from or do not know the names of your ancestors. Noticing is about feeling and sensing, not overthinking.*[86]

Personally, my lineage includes my friends, boyfriends, and students who died of AIDS. My yoga teaching grew out of my AIDS activism, and it was clear from the start that my community was struggling with the trauma of the AIDS epidemic. We were facing illness, death, and grief. Trauma is what brought me back to yoga in my early twenties, and I know it's what brings so many people to yoga. So, trauma isn't so much an obstacle to yoga, but a doorway. It's an entry point for so many of us, and the way we are greeted at that door will dictate whether we embrace the practice or walk away because we don't feel welcome or safe.

It's important to differentiate trauma-sensitive yoga from yoga therapy for people with PTSD or other diagnosed mental health conditions. Most yoga teachers aren't trained in treating medical conditions, and it's outside of their scope of practice. If students have a diagnosed condition that they are seeking support with, then it's best if they find a teacher or therapist who has training in that area.

Cultivating Safety

We need to challenge the traditional yoga class structure and find ways to elevate each student's ability to sense what they need at any given moment. This is important because trauma can take away our agency and trigger the fight or flight or freeze and fawn nervous system response. In the end, our goal is to support people in regaining a sense of control. This means giving them tools to begin to turn their awareness within, at their own pace, and in ways that feel safe. This can look like a lot of different things in yoga practice. For some people, it can mean simply finding different variations of a pose, or skipping a subtle practice that feels too interior-focused.

The point is that there isn't a prescriptive way to approach trauma-sensitive teaching. Different people have different triggers, but there are some general things we can do to support a slow and safe reconnection with the body. For example, we can avoid telling people what their experience should be. If I say, "This pranayama practice is very calming." But, a student doing the practice starts to feel anxious, does that invalidate their experience?

Trauma-sensitive teaching requires heightened awareness on your part. This includes awareness of your own positionality and privileged identities, that way you can be aware of what you're bringing into the room. Understanding who you are allows you to respect the fact that other people have very different experiences than you do. Making space for those experiences can be one of the most healing practices we can provide.

As Nityda Gessel explained in the opening quote for this chapter, working on yourself also allows for the potential of co-regulation. That means you can be an example of a regulated nervous system, even if there are challenges happening. You can teach by example, which in the end, is the most powerful way to teach.

Although interoception may be one of the goals of yoga, it's trauma-sensitive to focus primarily on grounding practices, such as bringing awareness to what students are experiencing through their senses, rather than turning inward to sensations of the breath, or watching the mind. That turning inward can be taught slowly over time, when the students feel ready. Even though I love teaching pranayama, yoga nidra, and meditation, I also recognize that those can be the most challenging practices of yoga. Sometimes focusing on asana can actually be more accessible if your students are dealing with trauma.

There isn't a list of poses or practices that are specifically trauma informed, since it's more about the way they are taught. But, there may be poses that are triggering depending on the community you are working with. For example, if you have students who may have experienced sexual trauma, you would want to avoid sexually suggestive poses, or poses where the body is very exposed. If you're working with incarcerated populations, you would want to avoid having students put their hands behind their head, or face a wall.

Most of all, it's important to remember that it's not your job to be a therapist, and you don't want to purposely trigger students. But, if it happens unintentionally, it's important to give students support, which can look like talking with them after class or providing additional resources and referrals. Giving the option to leave class early is also helpful. Remember your scope of practice, and be sure to have clear boundaries regarding what you can and can't address with your students. Of course, if you are interested in supporting people with trauma it can be very helpful to pursue further training in this area.

Scenario

You notice that one student is giving another student a lot of attention. Let's call them John and Bill. John is a longtime student, and Bill has recently joined your in-person class. John is acting like a quasi-teacher by bringing Bill props and giving him some pointers during the class. What do you do?

Response

Over the years, the most challenging situations I have faced in my yoga classes have been conflicts between students. Sometimes students will argue over a certain spot in the classroom, or they'll argue about the room being too hot or too cold, wanting to open or close windows, etc. Sometimes the situation gets worse and becomes a form of harassment, which I've also seen.

In this situation between Bill and John, I would get involved immediately. First, I could redirect John and ask him and the other students to focus on themselves and use this time to do their personal practice, which is internal. If the situation persists, I would approach John after class and ask him to allow me to be the teacher, and to give other students the space to have their own practice.

There's also an opportunity here to encourage John to take yoga teacher training himself. Maybe this is his way to show you that he wants to be a teacher.

Further Reflection

- What is your relationship with your own trauma, and how does that impact your teaching?

- In your personal practice can you integrate all aspects of your being—your humanity and spirituality?

- What is your experience with your teachers regarding your personal trauma? Have they been supportive of your healing?

- What else can you do to cultivate a sense of safety in your yoga classes?

CHAPTER TEN

TEACHING SHAVASANA

Shavasana is a symbol of rebirth. We exit our practice a lit-
tle differently than how we came in. Our yoga practice itself
is actually serving as a liminal space. This is something really
beautiful. Relaxation practices like yoga nidra and meditation
can serve as opportunities to really move through and connect
through the changes we experience in a very interesting way.

Something is ending and something new is beginning. So
we're in that space of possibility and uncertainty. I think that's
very much what our practice is about. The idea that our prac-
tice looks really different moment to moment. The way you
practiced yesterday is different than today, different than it'll
be tomorrow. Embracing that level of change.

Also understanding that what you were able to experience
on the mat, how you were able to approach the practice, is sim-
ply left where it is. We're moving out of that moment in a trans-
formational way. I think this is where we begin to connect to
the transformative nature of yoga. Once we move out of that
corpse pose, we're able to embody something a little different.
It's almost like leaving ourselves in a receptive place, for a level
of newness to emerge.

I would mainly say to be gentle with yourself in shavasana.
Be gentle with the process. I think that's my biggest piece of

advice. Simply acknowledging that you're going to approach the practice differently each time. Remember to be gentle with how you're showing up today, and be gentle with what showing up looks like in your future practices. I think that's the best way to approach your practice with a little bit more intentionality.

—Shawn Moore

IT'S HARD TO EXPRESS the beauty you get to experience when teaching yoga. Although that beauty is not what other people may think it is. It's not the thrill of seeing people achieve greatness with their physical abilities like challenging forearm stands or backbends. For me, the joy of teaching often arises during the final relaxation at the end of a class, when I have a felt-sense of the beauty around me.

During that stillness, I often feel connected to my students in a way that transcends words. I look over them the way I would gaze at my garden and its beautiful flowers, with a sense of admiration and a feeling of responsibility and protection. There's an aliveness in my garden that I can also feel in that quiet yoga room when everyone has let down their guard and softened into a chair or the floor, allowing the earth to hold them.

It's easy to ignore the fact that shavasana means corpse pose, and sometimes I avoid calling it that in an effort to be trauma-sensitive. But as teachers, it's important to remember that at its core, shavasana is a practice of death. That isn't the end of the story. The death that shavasana represents is like the rebirth of a compost pile. Compost is magic. Dead leaves, stems, and old rotten roots are transformed into fresh earth through the heat of those tiny microbial life forms. In our practice, we turn the compost over and over. The heat, *tapas*, of our asana and pranayama practice transforms our thoughts and emotions so that in shavasana fresh sweet smelling soil can be produced.

The combination of heat, darkness, and stillness allows for something new to be born. So much can come from that new dirt. Food, flowers, and giant trees can grow from that new fruitful soil, if it's allowed to rest in a compost pile. Death offers so much potential for new growth and every shavasana allows for that possibility as well.

The thing that no one tells you about yoga is that it's not about looking better or feeling better, although those are great too. Yoga is about preparing for death. Yoga is a spiritual practice that is teaching us how to be in touch with our essence—the truth of our existence beyond this body and mind. The practices of yoga are meant to reveal our basic ignorance about who we are.

Patanjali says that the final obstacle, *klesha*, to our enlightenment is *abhinivesha*, the fear of death. When I'm teaching, I often ask my students how many of them think about death on a regular basis. Usually half the class raises their hands and the other half looks at me slightly concerned. So for the half of you who think about their death on a regular basis, it should come as no surprise that yoga is about becoming comfortable with the reality of our limited human existence, and connecting to the expansiveness of our spiritual nature.

For those of you who never think about death, you're probably going to stop reading this right here. But if you got this far, I just want to say thank you for being open to considering the ways that the limitations of the body and mind could actually support you in cultivating a more joyful and peaceful way of being in this world.

Reflection

What is your relationship with death? Can you find a way to contemplate it in your practice?

A Conversation with Death

If we look back at the most ancient yoga teachings that we have access to, we find that there is a theme of death and spirituality. *The Katha Upanishad* from 900 BCE is a conversation between Yama, the god of death, and Nachiketa, a young boy. This also happens to be the text with the earliest reference to yoga.

In the story, Nachiketa's father announces that he is a devoted spiritual practitioner and is giving away all his possessions. But Nachiketa notices that his father only gives away the worst of his possessions. He gives away all his old cows that no longer give milk and other things that he doesn't need or use. So, Nachiketa questions his father about this, and asks why he isn't giving away his most precious possessions.

Nachiketa's father reacts by getting very angry, and in the spirit of giving away his sacred possessions, he proclaims, "To Death I give you!"[87] With that Nachiketa is sent to Yama, the god of death's, house. Unfortunately, Yama isn't home, so Nachiketa sits outside his door patiently waiting for three days and three nights. When Yama comes back, he's embarrassed to have kept Nachiketa waiting because the young boy is a member of a high caste.

This brings up an important point, which I've only touched on briefly. We need to recognize the role of caste within the yoga teachings and how caste has made yoga inaccessible for so many people. For more information, check out the work of Equality Labs, an organization working to address caste in modern society.[88]

After returning to find Nachiketa waiting, Yama says, "Well, because I made you wait for three days, I'm going to give you three wishes." Nachiketa's first wish is for his father to accept him back. His second wish is to have a fire ceremony named for him. The third thing that Nachiketa asks for is to know the secret of death, and to know what happens when we die. Yama tries to convince him to ask for something else, but upon recognizing that he is an intelligent and thoughtful child, he finally gives in and teaches Nachiketa the secret of death:

> *The all-knowing Self was never born,*
> *Nor will it die. Beyond cause and effect,*
> *This Self is eternal and immutable.*
> *When the body dies, the Self does not die.*
>
> *When the wise realize the Self,*
> *Formless in the midst of forms, changeless*
> *In the midst of change, omnipresent*
> *And supreme, they go beyond sorrow.*[89]

Pratyahara

Some people say that shavasana is the most challenging yoga pose—and in many ways that's true. In my experience, it's incredibly hard to put down my phone, turn my awareness within, and be with the chaos and clutter in my mind. And, I've been practicing for over 30 years! For new students this can be a very big ask.

Shavasana is a practice of *pratyahara*, sense withdrawal, which is the fifth limb of Patanjali's ashtanga yoga. Sense withdrawal is a key transitional step in all meditative practices. It's turning your awareness from outer to inner. Rather than focusing on what you're experiencing through your senses, what you see, hear, touch, etc., you turn inward. This could include awareness of emotions, thoughts, breath, heartbeat, internal organs, energy, etc.

Pratyahara is a combination of interoception and embodiment. It's only when we're inwardly focused that we are truly in our bodies. This step back into ourselves can be challenging, especially if we're dealing with trauma, anxiety, or any mental health concerns—which most of us are. Research shows that a third of all adults in the U.S. are experiencing anxiety and depression, and for young adults between the age of eighteen to twenty-four, the number is up to nearly half.[90]

As a teacher, I've learned to be patient with my students in regard to pratyahara. I don't expect someone who has spent their life outwardly focused to be able to quickly turn within. Of course, some people can do it instinctively, which is amazing, but many of them struggle with this redirected attention. What I find helpful is clear instruction and active practices that draw the attention inward. What does not seem very helpful are long periods of total silence or vague generalizations about being mindful. (I provide examples of pratyahara practices that are more active at the end of this chapter.)

Shavasana's dark, quiet, safe place is also a space where our feelings can become untangled from each other and from our knotted thoughts. There's a release that is not only physical, but also emotional and mental. We can create space between thoughts, space between feelings, and space between thoughts and feelings.

It reminds me of the transformation of a caterpillar into a butterfly. Shavasana is like the chrysalis stage where the caterpillar tucks itself into a cocoon and hibernates. In that safe, dark space it's body literally turns to mush and transforms into a new version of itself. It grows wings, often with bright colors and patterns, and when it finally emerges from the cocoon, it can fly.

Yoga Nidra

It's helpful to differentiate between shavasana, the physical posture, and yoga nidra, the guided meditation practice that we can do in that posture. There are many different forms of yoga nidra, which may include moving awareness around the body, progressive relaxation techniques, imagery, affirmations, and meditation.

Sometimes yoga nidra is treated as an extended practice of shavasana. But it's really much more. Indu Arora, explains that, "Yoga

nidra as an advanced form of meditation that bridges the gap between meditation and samadhi."[91]

Many forms of yoga nidra rely on the panchamaya kosha model,
which I discussed on page 157. This model is based on interconn-
nectedness. That means that our thoughts affect our energy, which
in turn affects our physical body. There is no separateness. Additionally, the subtler layers are actually more influential. So, thoughts and
emotions have tremendous influence over the body.

When teaching shavasana, or a longer yoga nidra session, it's useful to spend extra time making sure students are very comfortable.
Offering additional props, usually under the neck and knees, can be
really helpful, as can a blanket and an eye pillow. On the mat, help
students find a position for their arms that they can hold comfortably.

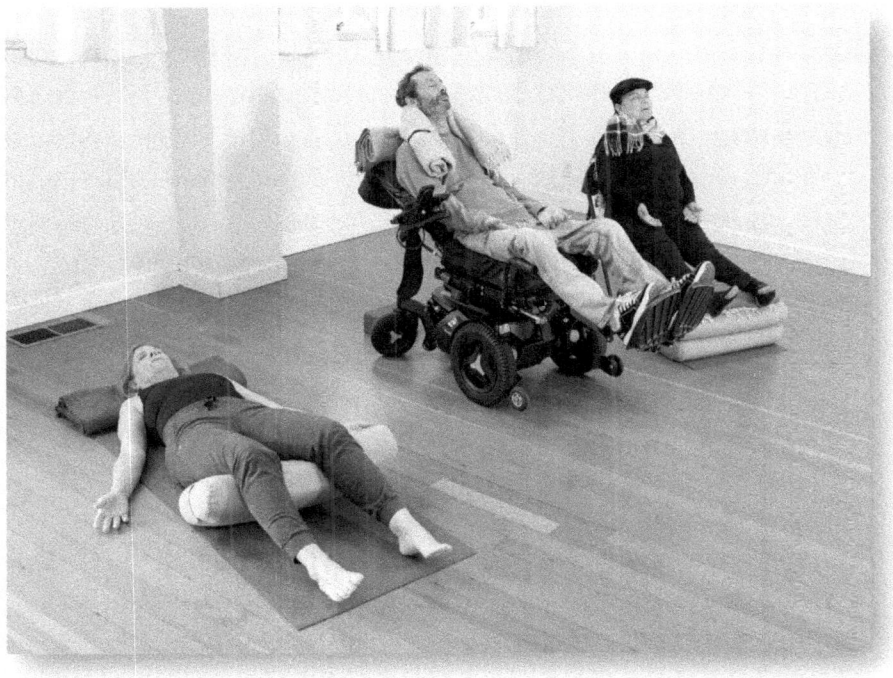

Three students practicing shavasana, *corpse pose. The student in the middle
is using a rolled blanket as a neck support, and they are all using a variety
of props to support the body in this resting pose.*

Sometimes, small supports under the back of the wrists can help. Offering alternative positions for shavasana, such as sitting up, or lying on the side, can also make the practice more accessible.

In a chair, it can be challenging to get comfortable for shavasana. Chair yoga students may benefit from neck support and elevating the feet and legs if possible. I often have to help students individually in order to find a position that they can hold for an extended period of time without straining or potentially falling out of the chair, which I've had happen in my classes.

Practice Ideas

Body Scan

Encourage students to bring a neutral awareness to their body and to notice their body without bringing in any judgments about it—accepting it for exactly how it is right now. Ask them to move their awareness from feet to head or head to feet, spending as much time as they want exploring sensation and energy, and to continually remind themselves to be neutral and accepting. If possible, encourage them to bring loving kindness to their body, thanking it for doing all the things it does.

Panchamaya Kosha—The 5 Bodies

Yoga nidra can be a journey through the panchamaya kosha. In practice, you would guide students to move from gross to subtle. First experiencing their physical body, *annamaya kosha*, which could include tensing and relaxing their body or doing a body scan. Then bring awareness to their *pranamaya kosha*, the energy body, noticing their breath or energy moving. Then *manomaya kosha*, the mental body, noticing the thoughts in their mind. Then, *vijnanamaya kosha*, the intuitive body, watching and observing their body, breath, and mind. Lastly, *anandamaya kosha*, the bliss body, experiencing a sense of bliss, relief, relaxation or whatever they find there. You can also remind them that beneath all the koshas is the *Atman* itself, pure consciousness.

Earth's Embrace

Ask students to notice the parts of their body that are touching the floor or chair. Guide them to become aware of the earth below them, and the eternal force of gravity pulling their body into the earth. As they exhale, ask them to see if they can relax into the pull of gravity, allowing their body to feel heavy. Invite them to release any tension or stress into the earth—to feel it pouring out and down into the earth itself. Ask them to imagine gravity as an embrace or hug from Mother Earth, holding them tightly.

Light & Energy

I avoid using any specific imagery for my students since it might be triggering, but general imagery of light and energy feels more neutral and accessible. You can guide students to choose their own color of light, and to decide whether they prefer it to be warm or cool. They can imagine the light or energy coming in from the top of their head and filling their body, or focus the light or energy in a specific place in their body that needs healing.

Choose Your Own Healing Journey

Imagery is a powerful healing tool that can be of tremendous benefit when incorporated in guided relaxation or yoga nidra practice. But it can be harmful to use imagery in a group yoga class when you don't really know your students' trauma history or have a chance to work with them individually to explore what kind of imagery might be most helpful.

For example, I once led a yoga nidra practice and talked about, "waves of relaxation moving through the body." At the end of the class a student came up to me and said she felt seasick from imagining the waves. That showed me how careful I need to be with what may seem like neutral images to me.

Instead, what can work well is to guide students to choose their own healing imagery. There are many ways to do this. One, as described in the section above, might include choosing a color of light or energy. A more detailed way to use imagery is to lead your students on a healing journey where they are choosing everything along the way, and where they have control. Here's a sample of what that might look like:

Find a position where your body is comfortable, cover yourself so that you'll stay warm, and cover your eyes if you want. I'll offer some prompts for a personal healing journey, and you're welcome to stop at any time.

Think of a place where you feel really comfortable and relaxed. It could be in a park, on a beach, or in your own living room. Once you've chosen a place, begin to look around with your mind's eye. Notice the colors, listen to sounds, feel the textures, smell the smells.

Then think of someone you love and admire and invite them to come visit you in this place. Invite this special person to come sit with you, and then ask them a question. It can be any question you want. Maybe something like, "What do I need for my healing and growth?" Then listen for an answer. Whenever you're ready, thank them for coming to visit you.

Look around your space one last time, and remember that this place is always there for you. Bring your awareness back to your breath, and slowly come back. Opening your eyes if they were closed. Look around and connect with your surroundings. Take a moment to think of your special place, and know that it's always there for you no matter what is happening or where you are.

Scenario

You're teaching an in-person yoga class and during shavasana a student is snoring loudly and disturbing the other students.

Response

This is a relatively common occurrence in most yoga classes, and it can be surprisingly difficult to respond to. You need to find a way to address this without further disturbing the other students, or scaring the student who is asleep. You also need to be careful about not using touch since the student is unconscious and can't give you consent to touch them.

It may sound strange, but the first thing I do is send a mental message to that student to breathe more deeply. If that doesn't work, I sit next to them and breathe a little more deeply myself. If that still doesn't work, I whisper something to them. If I know their name, I'll say their name, and "You're snoring." I might also say, "Can you roll to your side for the rest of the practice?" Because that will prevent them from snoring further.

In fact, the best way to handle this situation is to prevent it from occurring. If someone knows they have a tendency to snore, ask them to prop their head up higher with more support, such as in an inclined shavasana with a bolster behind their back. Or ask them to practice on their side. A side-lying shavasana can be very comfortable with support under the head and between the legs. They can also have an additional support in front of them, like a bolster, which they can hug.

Further Reflection

• How do your feelings about death impact the way you teach yoga?

• Do you do shavasana in your personal practice?

• What is your experience of pratyahara?

• What is your favorite form of yoga nidra?

CHAPTER ELEVEN

TEACHING PRANAYAMA

To make pranayama accessible, it's important to remember that you don't have to do fancy breath retention, or so-called "advanced practices." If the students are working on getting comfortable with their breathing, or getting an awareness of their breath, that alone is a really simple yet profound accessible pranayama practice. You're teaching people a way to take some of the pressure off of themselves.

Thinking about working with the breath as a progression rather than an isolated pranayama practice is also helpful. To start very simply and allow students to take their time with each step of a breath practice in order to actually get integrated and settled before adding on.

You can also invite students to try pranayama in different positions, different orientations, so they get a sense of how to experience spaciousness in their breath. Where do they get the most room to breathe? And giving students the opportunity to actually figure that out for themselves on that given day is important.

Then when they do the entire pranayama practice, say, at the end of class, the students will already understand that they get to choose what position to do the pranayama practice in. They'll already know for themselves how to prioritize spaciousness and capacity for their breath and then adjust accordingly. There's a balance between offering enough space for students to establish agency and have their own experience and also giving enough structure so that they don't feel like you're sending them out in the ocean in a boat without a sail.

—Melissa Shah

IN ONE OF THE MOST poetic passages of his Yoga Sutras, Patanjali explains that pranayama, the breathing practices, allow our inner light, or spirit, to shine. He says, "As a result [of pranayama] the veil over the inner Light is destroyed."[92] This sutra conveys the potency of pranayama to help us awaken. But what's so poignant about this particular sutra is that it uses powerful figurative language to convey Patanjali's basic message: We are light—Purusha, interconnected spiritual beings—and the yoga practices help us to remove the veil, or the obstacles, to experiencing that truth.

In the beginning of this same chapter, *Sadhana Pada*, the portion on practice, Patanjali identifies the main obstacles to our self-realization or enlightenment, which he refers to as the five *klesha*. The klesha begin with one fundamental issue, the ignorance of our spiritual nature, which Patanjali calls *avidya*.

Avidya is a state of confusion. We have identified with the body and mind and believe that they are who we really are. At the same time, we think that spirit is an illusion. The yoga teachings posit that we are spirit, immortal and permanent, rather than body and mind, which are mortal and impermanent. According to sutra 2.5, "Ignorance is regarding the impermanent as permanent, the impure as pure, the painful as pleasant, and the non-Self as the Self."[93]

Overcoming avidya is truly the goal of yoga, but this shift in identification can feel impossible and confusing. How amazing it is to realize that the basic tools of yoga can support us in correcting this confusion. In particular, working with the breath gives us such an accessible and practical way to expand into this deeper understanding of who we are. Pranayama has the power to not only destroy the veil over our inner light, but to allow us to shift our sense of self—to realize we are that light, that spirit. This reminds me of a famous quote from the Indian poet Kabir. He answers the timeless question, "What is God?" by explaining, "It is the breath inside the breath."[94]

Three Pathways to Practice: Body, Breath, and Mind

Today, we often perceive separation between the body, breath, and mind, as if they are truly distinct from each other. Instead, it could be helpful to conceive of them as different vibrational levels of the same thing. A helpful analogy is ice, water, and steam. Are they different things? Ice, water, and steam are all different vibrational forms of H_2O. They're the same, but also different.

When I move my body in asana it automatically impacts my breath and my mind. When I do breathing practices, it shifts my body and my mind. When I meditate, it changes my breath and my body. These three layers—body, breath, and mind—are inseparable elements of our embodied human experience. This understanding is essential when working to make yoga more accessible because it provides us three distinct pathways to practice.

As I mentioned previously on page 180, if a particular asana isn't accessible for someone, they can visualize the practice in their mind, or move the breath the way it might move in that pose. On the other hand, if someone is struggling with trauma or anxiety, or if they are neurodivergent, working directly with the mind or the breath might feel overwhelming. In that case, focusing on the body can be more accessible. Practicing more asana and less subtle practices might be the best choice.

The idea of three paths to practice—body, breath, and mind—reminds me of getting directions from Google Maps on my phone.

Once I put in my destination, I can decide if I want to drive, walk, take transit, cycle, or rideshare, and that answer depends a lot on my capacity at that moment. These five options are all different, but they will take me to the same destination. In the same way, students can choose to engage their body with asana, their breath with pranayama, or their mind with meditation based on what feels most comfortable to them.

I remember one student who was a young man in his twenties who had previously been very healthy, and all of a sudden he found himself dealing with some kind of serious chronic illness that doctors couldn't diagnose. He was struggling with this new disability, especially at such a young age. He came to me for private yoga therapy sessions, and it was challenging for me to find practices that he enjoyed. He had such extreme fatigue, that everything I asked him to do felt like a chore.

In particular, he was having trouble breathing and was often short of breath. One day, I decided to lead a chant, and asked him to follow along. Instead of his normal strained breath, he let out this strong and powerful singing voice that really shocked me. I asked in amazement, "Where did that come from?" He smiled broadly and explained that he used to be in a choir, and that he loved to sing. That helped me realize that singing and chanting would be the most effective practice for him. So, we ended up spending a good portion of our sessions chanting together, and I could see that he felt some freedom in those moments.

Trauma-Sensitive Pranayama

Pranayama are subtle practices which can take patience and perseverance, yet they offer profound benefits including calming the mind and reducing stress. Luckily, these powerful practices are available to anyone who is breathing. Although, not everyone needs to practice them. There are a variety of reasons why a pranayama practice might not be appropriate for someone. Some pranayama practices can bring up stored emotions and trauma and can potentially exacerbate mental health issues such as anxiety. This is especially true for practices that move a lot of energy such as *deergha swasam*, deep breathing, *kapalabhati*, skull shining breath, as well as *bhastrika*, bellows breath.

There are many valid reasons why someone wouldn't want to do pranayama, and it's important to support all students in finding their own way into the subtle practices of yoga. So, I try to be encouraging and enthusiastic without being overbearing. I find it helps to use a positive approach. I always tell my students, "If you're breathing, you're doing it right!" Starting with this affirmation can completely shift our experience of breathing practices. Plus, it's true. If you're alive you have figured out how to breathe. On the other hand, starting with the thought that you're breathing wrong can make pranayama very uncomfortable and ineffective. It can create additional anxiety and tension in the practice, and create the opposite effect than we're seeking.

Unfortunately, most people come to yoga with this idea that they need to be fixed, or that they're not good enough. Those ideas may inspire them to practice, but they can quickly lead to frustration when change doesn't happen or if practice feels challenging. It's also not true. We're all doing the best we can with what we have. Even trauma responses are effective and intelligent. They are the body, mind, and nervous system responding the best way they know how under pain and pressure. Trauma responses often keep us alive, and that should be celebrated instead of denigrated. According to Nityda Gessel:

Pain and trauma do not halt our personal evolution or spiritual progression. They provide us an opportunity to wake up all the more... The thought of being with pain, memory, and leftover trauma stored in the body can feel scary or overwhelming, but there is a way to do this that is compassionate and that works with the pace of each unique nervous system. Lifting the veil happens gradually, over time. Awakening, the process of seeing clearly again, of returning to our true nature, is skillful and sacred—not to be rushed. It's liberative.[95]

Start with Exploration

Let your students spend time appreciating their breath, and noticing its nuances. Let them use their interceptive skills before changing or manipulating the breath. It can be incredibly effective to observe the breath without changing it. It's a chance to learn about subtlety, especially for students who come to yoga for the big sensations of physical practices. It can be a major shift to focus on the details of the breath. It might feel challenging in a new way, and even feel overwhelming and confusing to spend time simply observing.

These are powerful practices that need to be taken seriously, and before students begin, they should understand what they're working with. You could consider this the intake phase, gathering information, both for you and for the students.

If observation feels comfortable, students can begin to slowly shift or alter their breath. This could mean deepening it slightly by changing where they feel the breath in the body, or it could mean lengthening or slowing the breath. It's helpful to pause after every pranayama practice and ask students to notice how they feel, or to notice the effects of the practice. Eventually, students can become aware of the ways that changing the breath can impact their nervous system and energy.

Students can explore the different effects of lengthening their inhale or their exhale. Melissa Shah describes these aspects of the practice according to ayurveda, with the terms *brahmana* and *langhana*. Brahmana means expansion and is used to describe an energizing practice where you increase the inhalation. Langhana means reduction, and refers to a calming practice that comes from lengthening the exhalation.

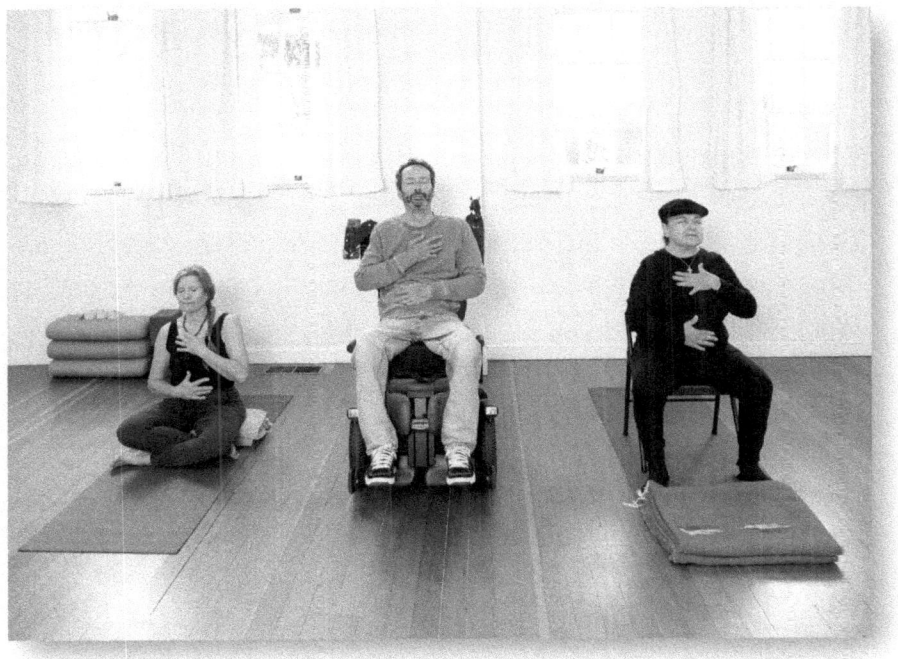

Students with one hand on their belly and one on their chest noticing their breath

Permission to Stop

For your students, it can be helpful to know that they can always come back to the initial stage of exploration without manipulation. It's so helpful to remind them that they have choice and control. This is as simple as telling the students they're always free to stop if something is uncomfortable. I can tell you from personal experience, as someone who has anxiety, that breathing practices are sometimes triggering. So proceed with awareness and gentleness.

I like to refer to this as a disclaimer that I share at the beginning of every pranayama practice I lead. It can also be repeated later during the practice, but it's an essential opening remark. Something like, "Remember, if you feel uncomfortable at any time, you're welcome to stop practicing and relax or observe the breath."

Bigger isn't Better

This idea that bigger isn't better when it comes to pranayama is something that took me years to figure out for myself. I always thought that more was better, and that the deeper my breath, the more advanced I was becoming. But that just isn't true. In pranayama, we get to focus on subtle and slow rather than on big and loud. Deep breaths are not necessarily what we need. In fact, constantly telling people, "Just take a deep breath," ignores the fact that deep breaths are not always accessible for people, or that helpful.

Also, the eventual goal of pranayama is actually stillness and quietness, so deep breathing isn't necessary to reach that goal. Shifting this understanding can change the way you teach the practice and remove the goal-orientation that is so common in contemporary yoga. I'll describe some specific practices below that lend themselves to subtle and slow breathing.

Avoid Retention

Many yoga teachers instruct breath retention, holding the breath in or out, for beginning practitioners, but I think that's too much too fast. In fact, it reminds me of something I learned from Nityda Gessel, who I quoted earlier. In general, she defines trauma as either too much too fast, or too little for too long. I think it's important to allow students time to get comfortable with pranayama before practicing retention—potentially a lot of time! I don't like to classify practices as beginner or advanced, but this is one exception to my rule. Retention is a practice for experienced students who have a good sense of their breath and how changing it impacts their mind and their nervous system.

Instead, work on momentary pauses, and notice how they feel. Increase those pauses slowly rather than holding the breath for a particular count. That's the other thing: Not only would I avoid teaching retention to new or relatively new students, I would avoid instructing pranayama practices with specific counts all together. This is an external control on the students' breath, and it feels like an overreach in group yoga classes.

An example of where I see this happening is in practices like *sama vritti*, which means equal breathing or box breathing.[96] In this practice, students are asked to inhale for four seconds, hold the breath for four seconds, exhale for four seconds, and hold the breath out for four seconds. There's also a similar 4, 7, 8 breathing practice that's getting a lot of media attention these days,[97] which includes inhaling for four seconds, holding the breath for seven seconds, and exhaling for eight seconds. That's a long retention for someone who doesn't have an established pranayama practice.

There is a variation of sama vritti, where you make the inhalation and exhalation the same length and don't retain the breath. That is more appropriate for beginners, and can be made more accessible by simply allowing students to control the length of their breath rather than telling them how long it should be.

For example, rather than saying, "Inhale for a count of four, and exhale for a count of four." You could say, "Begin to count the length of your gentle slow breath. Count the inhale and count the exhale. See if you can make them the same by shortening whichever one is longer." This approach allows students to find their own breathing speed even in a large group yoga class. It also furthers their interoceptive skills by asking them to count the length of their regular breathing rather than imposing a false "correct" length.

This is not to say that we should discourage retention and slowing the breath eventually, when a student is ready. It's just that I'm focusing on the most accessible and generally safe techniques here. Also, it's helpful to recognize that teaching some pranayama techniques requires special training, and I would encourage you to seek it out. If you haven't received that kind of training, I hope that what I'm suggesting here can support you in creating a safe and effective experience for both you and your students.

Sample Practices

Deergha Swasam—Deep Breathing

Deergha swasam, which means "deep breathing," is sometimes called yogic breathing, three-part breathing, or diaphragmatic breathing. It is a useful technique for becoming more conscious of how the breath is moving. It's generally taught as a way to deepen the breath, which is not always helpful. But you can make it a subtle practice of awareness.

Generally, this practice is taught as an inhale from the bottom up and an exhale from the top down. But some teachers use a slightly different order. The main goal is to engage the diaphragm muscle which is the largest and most efficient mover of the lungs. When breathing this way, you may feel your belly expand on the inhalation because as the diaphragm contracts it shortens and moves downward pulling the lungs down to expand them. With this downward movement the diaphragm presses on the top of the abdominal organs and displaces them forward. Then, as the diaphragm relaxes back up into the thoracic cavity, the abdominal organs move back into their relaxed position.

The relationship between the diaphragm and the other internal organs is very important because the diaphragm, and its constant rhythmic movement, are associated with moving lymph fluid, massaging the digestive organs and the heart, as well as other functions.[98] In fact, diaphragmatic breathing is associated with various health benefits such as reducing stress and anxiety, supporting people with lung diseases, and reducing blood pressure.[99] Recent research shows that slow, deep breathing may even prevent Alzheimer's disease.[100]

In this practice, students can place a hand on the belly and a hand on the chest, and notice where the body is moving when they breathe. If it's comfortable, students can deepen the breath by pulling in the abdomen slightly at the end of the exhale, and expanding it slightly on the inhale. Having a hand on the belly assists in increasing interoception. Similarly, one hand on the upper chest can be used to feel the inhale expand the chest all the way up to the collarbones.

Students can also move their hands to their side ribs to experience how the ribcage is moving. For many people, connecting with the movement in the lower ribs is more accessible than connecting with movement in the belly. The diaphragm is attached to the lower ribs in the front of the body, and to the spine in the back. The image of bucket handles moving up and down is often associated with the movement of the rib cage, with the ribs attached at the sternum and the spine. On the inhale, the ribs expand out and up on the sides and the diaphragm lowers. On the exhale, the ribs move down and in and the diaphragm relaxes.

To make the practice more accessible, deergha swasam can also be explored in a reclined shavasana. Students can place a hand or an object like a small sandbag or folded blanket on their belly and feel the movement there. Similarly, lying prone in crocodile pose can offer an opportunity to explore the movement of the belly against the floor in connection with the movement of the diaphragm.

Ujjayi—Whispering Breath

To help lengthen the breath, students can explore controlling the movement of the breath in the throat. This practice is called *ujjayi* (which literally means victorious breath, but is also called ocean breath or whispering breath) and is helpful for progressing in pranayama. To better understand this technique, students can pretend to clean a pair of eyeglasses as if they are fogging up the lenses by making a "haa" sound with the mouth open. Then have them close the mouth and make that same sound, which may sound like they're whispering.

This whispering, or wheezing sound, is the result of air passing through the reduced opening in the throat. Ujjayi is done by controlling the glottis which is the part of your throat that closes when you swallow. By reducing the size of the opening, the air takes longer to enter or leave the lungs, and the breath is lengthened.

I usually have students learn this technique on the exhalation first. They begin with a deep inhale with a relaxed throat. On the exhale, as they engage ujjayi, they can feel the breath leaving very slowly and smoothly with a whispering sound. With practice, ujjayi can be added to other pranayama techniques to lengthen the breath.

Nadi Shuddhi—Alternate Nostril Breath

Nadi shuddhi (also known as *nadi shodhana, sukha purvaka,* and *aniloma viloma*) means energy channel purification, and is also known as alternate nostril breathing. This practice balances energy on the right and left sides of the body, and that feeling of balance may be experienced as peacefulness in the mind.

Throughout the day, one nostril is usually more open than the other, and this nostril dominance switches every hour or so, back and forth. Traditionally, yogis found that dominance of one nostril would correspond to increased energy going to the opposite hemisphere of the brain.[101] With nadi shuddhi, the focus is on creating balance between the two hemispheres—and balance is another name for equilibrium and peace.

To practice nadi shuddhi, those who are comfortable using their right hand can make a gentle fist and extend the last two fingers and thumb. Bringing the hand to the nose, close the right nostril with the thumb and exhale from the left nostril. Inhale left, switch nostrils, and exhale right. Continue with this pattern of inhale, switch, exhale. Breathing gently and slowly.

Once the pattern is comfortable, students can lengthen the exhalation, using ujjayi breathing to control the breath and slow it down, eventually making the exhalation twice as long as the inhale. Be sure there is no straining or shortness of breath. If so, return the breath to normal.

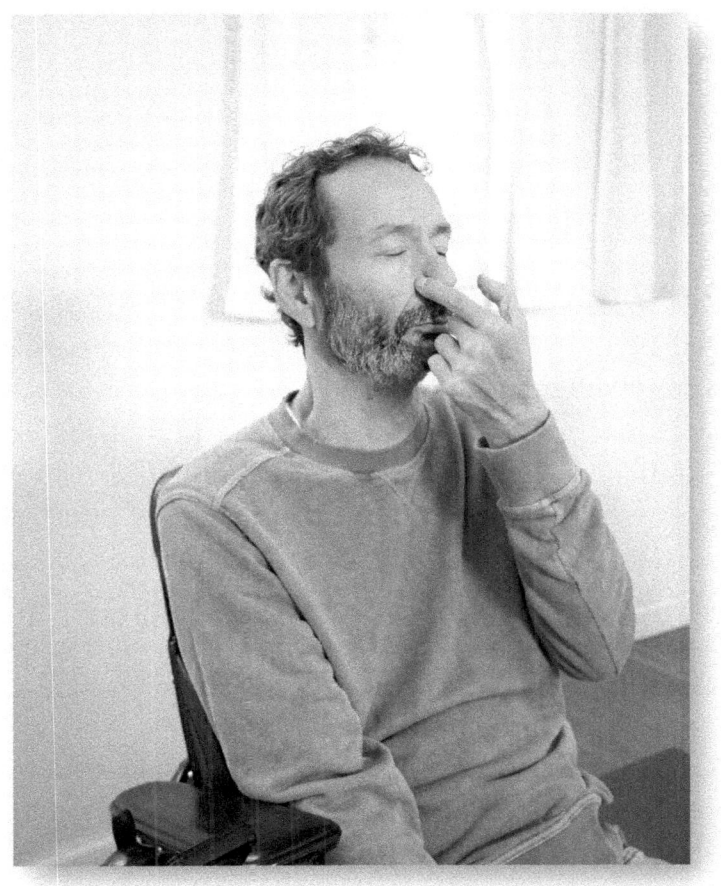

A student practicing alternate nostril breathing using a variation of the traditional hand position—the index finger and thumb of the left hand.

If using the right hand is not comfortable for students, the left can be used. Or, if the hand position is uncomfortable, students can use their index finger and thumb. Alternatively, if using the hand is not possible, the practice can be done just with the mind. Without using the hand, imagine the breath moving in the same pattern—out and in from one nostril at a time. This is actually a subtler form of the practice because it takes a lot of mental concentration to experience the movement of the breath, and to stay focused. Over time, the student may be able to follow the breath in this way and experience the movement of the breath in and out of each nostril.

After practicing nadi shuddhi, or any pranayama, it is useful to take a moment and have the students notice how they're feeling before moving on to the next practice.

Kapalabhati—Skull Shining Breath

Kapalabhati is sometimes known as the breath of fire because it helps to stimulate and raise prana in the body. In fact, kapalabhati literally means "skull shining" because the practice raises energy up into the head. This practice is generally considered contraindicated for people with high blood pressure, pregnant people, anyone who had recent surgery, people with IBS, Crohn's, acid reflux, hiatal hernia, or other digestive issues, and people with anxiety. Because this covers a very large percentage of the population, it may be best to only do gentle variations of kapalabhati, or only do this practice after students are already comfortable with the other pranayama techniques included here, or simply leave it out.

The practice is done by repeatedly making a forceful exhalation, followed by a relaxed inhalation. For a more accessible variation, students can practice with the mouth open. First, snap the abdomen in to exhale and make the sound, "ha!" To inhale, allow the breath to return naturally through the nose or mouth. Once students are comfortable, they can close the mouth and practice with the breath moving through the nose only.

The challenge of this practice is to keep the diaphragm muscle relaxed the whole time, and allow the muscular action to come from the abdominal muscles instead. In the beginning, practice ten or fewer breaths per round, with only two or three rounds total. Over time students can increase the breaths per round according to their comfort level. Be sure there is no straining or shortness of breath.

The most important part of the practice is the final breath at the end of the practice. So, after the series of rapid breaths, exhale deeply, inhale using deergha swasam. Pause for a moment after the inhale, and then exhale very slowly. During this final exhalation the focus is on energy rising up the spine. If students feel lightheaded or any discomfort, they can return their breathing to normal. More experienced students, who are comfortable with kapalabhati, can experiment with using ujjayi during the final exhalation to slow the breath and focus on energy rising.

Scenario

A student comes up to you after class and says, "I really just come here to get stronger and more flexible. Do you mind if I leave before you do the breathing at the end of class? I find that part really boring."

This is a hard question to answer, not because students shouldn't be able to leave when they want to, but because I wouldn't want this student to disturb the other students when they are practicing pranayama. I might take this question as an opportunity for some education, and perhaps refer the student to some research on the physiological benefits of pranayama. For example, there's research that shows that pranayama can reduce blood pressure and stress and improve sleep quality[102]. It's also been shown to help support people with anxiety,[103] respiratory issues, cancer, and cardiovascular disease.[104]

I would hope that if this student was interested in getting stronger and more flexible, they may also want to support their health in ways that pranayama could help. (And pranayama may actually support them in getting stronger, because it can increase cardiovascular health among other things!)

On the other hand, boredom in pranayama can be a sign of trauma, and it's important that people honor their limits. So in the end, I think I would talk to this student about the health benefits of pranayama and of course allow them to leave. But, I would also share my concerns about how their leaving class early might disrupt the other students.

Further Reflection

• What is my experience of the breath in yoga?

• What is the biggest challenge in my personal pranayama practice?

• Can I find a way to help students celebrate their breath before changing it with these practices?

• What is my experience of retention in pranayama?

CHAPTER TWELVE

TEACHING MEDITATION

I like to think about meditation as a state of grace, something that descends. It's not something that we can actually make happen, no matter how "perfect" we think the posture is, or how advanced we think our technique is. All we're doing is preparing. I think we can allow people to tune into this idea that we're just preparing for that moment, where something that I experience as grace, just drops in. If all we're doing is preparing, it takes away any kind of constriction, expectation, performance of what it means to meditate.

Often, someone who is a beginner at meditation may have the most sublime, profound experiences. Because there's no expectation, there's no hierarchy in the practice. It's just, "Oh, here's my experience. It's like, wow, this is incredible." Not only did I have this sublime, profound experience, but my ability to articulate what transpired for me, is also a transmission. This is how someone who is a "beginner" is able to transmit the experience.

Every meditation or quiet moment that you have, including practicing the yamas and niyamas, is the preparation. Even if you think, "Yesterday, I didn't have a blissful, sublime amazing experience in my meditation." Even if it was very distracted and chaotic in some way, that meditation was still a preparation.

A lot of times we tend to want to grade our experiences. We want to say, "Oh, I had a bad meditation today." No, you didn't. You had a practice that is creating a cumulative effect, not only on your nervous system, but on your entire practice. If I'm devoted to my practice, that devotion really makes it beautiful for me to keep unfolding and learning and deepening. But if I feel like I'm trying to get something, then it's a never ending journey of extraction, expectation, and comparison—all of the qualities of gripping that our practice can help us soften. Devotion inspires spaciousness and ease in our practice.

—Tracee Stanley

BEGINNING MEDITATORS often feel that they simply can't meditate because their minds are too busy. That is the universal experience of the mind; it's constantly jumping from thought to thought, frantically looking for ways to achieve happiness through the satisfaction of its desires. Of course, the mind's belief that happiness comes from outside of us is incorrect, and a major obstacle in itself. According to the yoga teachings, happiness and peace are the nature of our inner awareness. This is beautifully expressed in this section of the *Shvetashvatara Upanishad*:

It is the inner Self of all,
Hidden like a little flame in the heart.
Only by the stilled mind can It be known.
Those who realize It become immortal.

It is the blue bird; It is the green bird
With red eyes; It is the thundercloud,
And It is the seasons and the seas.
It has no beginning; It has no end.
It is the source from whom the worlds evolve.

From its divine power comes forth all this
Magical show of name and form, of you
And me, which casts the spell of pain and pleasure.
Only when we pierce through this magic veil
Do we see the One who appears as many?[105]

Meditation Education

In the classical yoga tradition, meditation is practiced by concentrating the mind on one thing—usually a Sanskrit mantra. Patanjali explains that concentration is the best way to remove the obstacles to our enlightenment. He says, "The practice of concentration on a single subject [or the use of one technique] is the best way to prevent the obstacles and their accompaniments."[106] He goes on to explain that we can cultivate this experience by, "Meditating on anything one chooses that is elevating."[107]

This traditional approach may not work for everyone, and there are many other ways to work with the mind. It may be helpful to explore different techniques and allow each student to discover which practice is the most comfortable for them. Different meditation techniques include grounding, focusing, mindfulness, body scans, imagery, visual meditation, and more. It can also mean using a combination of techniques at first, rather than just focusing on one thing.

It's important to teach meditation in a way that is inclusive and motivating rather than teaching in a way that might feel restrictive or exclusive. That may happen unconsciously if you are trained in a tradition that uses a specific form of meditation practice, or because you found a technique that works for you personally.

You can find this open-minded approach reflected in the Yoga Sutras. In chapter three, Patanjali explains that *dharana*, concentration, the sixth limb of ashtanga yoga, "Is the binding of the mind to one place, object, or idea."[108] It's an important definition, because he's focusing on the technique rather than on any specific object of concentration. In that way, he is opening the practice up to individual choice.

The Heart of Our Practice

In so many ways, meditation is the penultimate practice of yoga. It asks us to practice the core teaching of yoga: Quiet the mind to experience peace within. Remember Patanjali's famous sutra 1.2, *"yogas chitta vritti nirodhah,"* which means that stilling the mind is yoga. Meditation is an opportunity to go directly to the heart of what he's asking us to do.

So much of our yoga teaching tends to focus on asana that we tend to forget, or choose to ignore, the role of meditation. I think this is partially an element of contemporary yoga culture, but it could also be because meditation is challenging. Perhaps it's because of the subtlety of the practice, and how hard it can be to see progress. With asana, on the other hand, it's so easy to demonstrate the outward appearance of the practice. But, what would meditation look like on social media?

There are many benefits to meditation, including improved sleep quality, reduced anxiety and depression, boosted immune function, increased brain function, and lowered blood pressure, among others![109] The way for your students to tell if their meditation is working is that over a long period of time they notice a small shift. Maybe they feel a little more content, or less stressed. It can be subtle, but it's important for them to notice.

The thing is, I hardly know anyone who thinks they're very good at meditation. It often feels like a Sisyphean task. Constantly focusing the mind only to have it wander off feels like Sisyphus pushing that boulder up a hill only to have it roll back down again. We're sitting with our busy mind constantly trying to get it to calm down. But the thoughts keep coming and coming. The problem is that we conflate the ideal of meditation, a completely quiet mind, with the practice of it. As Tracee Stanley described above, we forget that there's tremendous benefit in the practice itself, even if we don't seem to be able to reach the final goal.

Trying to meditate reminds me of the way black flies get trapped inside my house. I'll often see a fly buzzing around my window, seemingly wanting to escape. Then I open the window to let it free, and somehow it always flies the wrong way and bangs itself into the glass, over and over again. It almost seems to want to stay inside. But when I do finally get the fly to escape through the open window, it quickly buzzes away, back into nature.

This is how my meditation often feels. It's like there's an opening right there, and so often I can't seem to reach it. Instead I just go back to the same thought and the same worries, over and over again. Sometimes, after sitting for a good period of time, my mind settles, and I find that opening to relaxation and to a moment of peace. It happens in a quick moment, and all of a sudden I feel free.

Stretching that fly analogy a little further, I often wonder where that fly came from, and how did it get inside my house? They just seem to appear from nothing. Just like my thoughts which seem to appear from nothing and return over and over. It reminds me of a powerful dialogue in the *Kena Upanishad* between a student and teacher that explores where the mind comes from:

The Student
Who makes my mind think?
Who fills my body with vitality?
Who causes my tongue to speak? Who is that
Invisible one who sees through my eyes
And hears through my ears?

The Teacher
The Self is the ear of the ear,
The eye of the eye, the mind of the mind,
The word of words, and the life of life.
Rising above the senses and the mind
And renouncing separate existence,
The wise realize the deathless Self.

It our eyes cannot see, nor words express;
It cannot be grasped even by the mind.
We do not know, we cannot understand,
Because It is different from the known
And It is different from the unknown.
Thus have we heard from the illumined ones.

That which makes the tongue speak but cannot be
Spoken by the tongue, know that as the Self.
This Self is not someone other than you.

That which makes the mind think but cannot be
Thought by the mind, that is the Self indeed.
This Self is not someone other than you.

That which makes the eye see but cannot be
Seen by the eye, that is the Self indeed.
This Self is not someone other than you.

That which makes the ear hear but cannot be
Heard by the ear, that is the Self indeed.
This Self is not someone other than you.

That which makes you draw breath but cannot be
Drawn by your breath, that is the Self indeed.
This Self is not someone other than you.[110]

Tools for Teaching Meditation

Like with everything else we teach, it's best to start at the beginning with our students and not assume that they have any previous knowledge or experience. In fact, I think one of the obstacles to people really learning about meditation is the incorrect information that they may have learned through the media.

We're led to think that meditation is sitting in total stillness without moving the body, and that the mind is completely peaceful with no thoughts interrupting us. This cliché is so far from the truth of the practice that it can interfere with the experience of students who really want to give meditation a try. The moment they're faced with their busy mind they think, "I can't meditate. My mind is too busy for this."

That also becomes a great excuse for a mind that isn't used to, and doesn't want, discipline. After a lifetime of doing whatever it wants, why would the mind want to be told what to do? Also, there are many real obstacles to meditation, such as neurodiversity and trauma, which impact the mind.

So rather than forcing people to sit in stillness for long periods of time, I think it's best to focus on education. The job of a yoga teacher includes educating your students about what meditation is—a practice that takes patience and lots of repetition. Explaining that during meditation the mind will wander—and that it's a normal part of the process—can take away a lot of shame and feelings of failure.

For beginners, it can be helpful to give clear instruction and teach an active practice such as observing the breath; repeating a mantra or word; a visual focus like a light, candle flame, or picture, or even a point on the floor in front of you; a mudra or gesture you make with your hand; or the use of mala beads or prayer beads (which I describe below).

It's also important to prioritize comfort, which means finding a position that doesn't create pain, and allowing students to move or change positions during meditation if they're uncomfortable. Sitting through the pain is not necessary. Instead, they can use their asana practice the way it was originally intended, as preparation for meditation. Remember that pranayama can help regulate the nervous system, which can make meditation much easier. Other subtle practices such as yoga nidra, chanting, prayer, and mudra also help support a meditation practice.

For many students, starting with long periods of silent meditation is not accessible and may actually be contraindicated. This is especially true for people with trauma or mental health issues such as depression.[111] It's important to start slowly with very short periods of silence to make sure the students are comfortable.

Also, offering multiple grounding points can be helpful. That could mean integrating a few different techniques into their practice such as simultaneously following the breath, repeating a mantra, and gazing at a spot on the floor. Or it could mean using mala beads, following the breath, and counting. The goal is to help students find a comfortable way into meditation that isn't overwhelming or too strict. That way they can slowly build a long term practice based on positive personal experiences with meditation.

I like to think of grounding points in meditation as being similar to the props we use in asana practice. Grounding points, like yoga props, are neutral, and whether or not to use them is an individual choice. As teachers, our job is simply to educate people about the different options they have in meditation, and as an Accessible Yoga instructor, our goal is to give people tools to make the practice as approachable as possible.

Generally, there are four categories of meditation techniques. Here are a few practices that fall within those categories:

1. Focusing: Using practices like mantra, breath, visual focus. This is the traditional technique of classical yoga.
2. Witnessing: Open awareness meditation and mindfulness meditation fall into this category. It includes practices such as

body scan, yoga nidra, making friends with the mind, and "yes" meditation, which I describe below. These approaches are non-directed and include observing the mind without focusing it.

3. Praying: This is any time you're speaking to the divine, your higher self, or God. An inner conversation which may include talking and/or listening.

4. Analyzing: "Who am I?" meditation. This is a technique of the Jnana Yoga tradition, where you ask yourself a series of questions and ponder them.

Sample Meditation Routine

The way I approach teaching meditation is to build toward it throughout the entire class. I usually spend the last few minutes educating the students about meditation specifically and then spend only a moment actually leading a meditation. After they've done the physical practices and shavasana, I ask the students to find a comfortable posture, whether it's sitting on the floor, sitting in a chair, or lying in bed. We then do some pranayama to prepare the nervous system and the mind for meditation.

Finally, I share some general guidance for silent meditation. Usually, I describe how to practice a particular form of meditation, such as repeating a mantra or observing the breath. I give students the option of using multiple grounding points, and keeping their eyes open if they prefer. I also make a point to say that it's normal for the mind to wander, and the practice of concentration is about noticing that it has wandered and gently bringing it back, again and again.

I keep the silent meditation to a maximum of one minute in public classes, unless I have been working with the students for a while. To be honest, I struggle with keeping those meditations so short, because with the energy of the group, I feel like I could sit for much longer. Group meditation has this powerful cumulative effect that can sweep along even those of us with very busy minds. But as the teacher, I need to keep part of my mind alert to what's happening in the room, and to the time.

Afterward, I end with a closing dedication. The dedication is an essential part of the practice where we commit the energy and peace that we found in our practice to either our own benefit, the benefit of others, or the entire universe. The dedication is a reminder of our interconnectedness, and also a way to make our practice a service to others.

Here's a sample meditation routine that I like to share with my students so they get a sense of what a personal meditation practice might look like. For a beginner practicing at home, this entire routine might be as short as five minutes or as long as fifteen. Generally, it's more helpful to do a shorter practice every day than a longer practice occasionally. That way meditation becomes an enjoyable habit and will have a bigger impact.

1. Check Your Posture. This could be sitting on the floor with props, in a chair, or lying in bed. Begin by bowing to yourself or to an altar with objects and images that are sacred to you.
2. Opening Centering. This could include chanting "Om" three times or chanting longer mantras if you know them.
3. Pranayama: This might include:
   - Deep breathing
   - Kapalabhati
   - Nadi Shuddhi
4. Silent Meditation: Use a specific technique or combination of techniques. Decide on the length of time beforehand and stick to that time. Don't overdo it.
5. Dedication: End with mantras or prayers to dedicate the benefits of your practice to yourself and others.

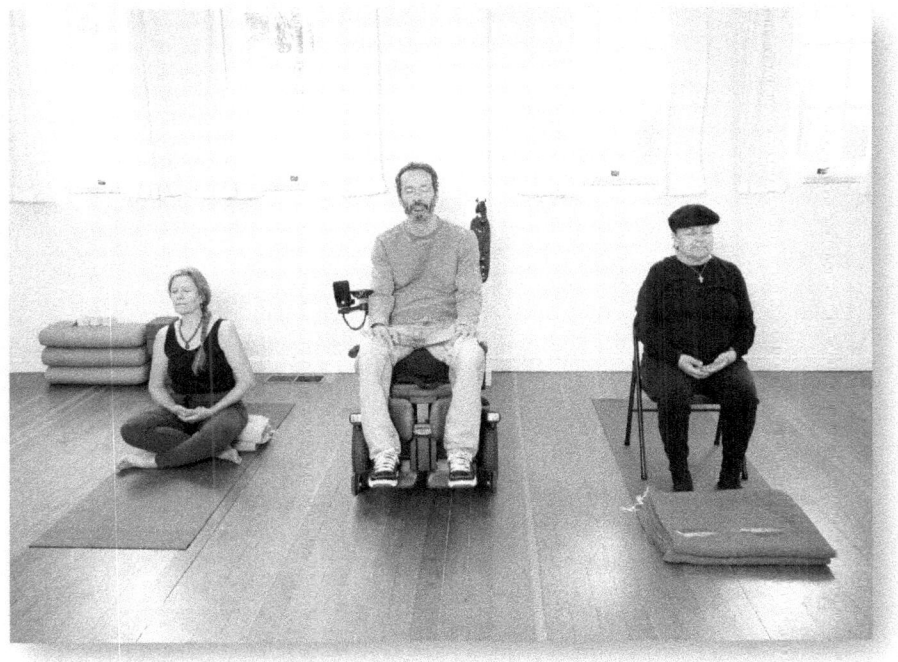

Students practicing meditation on a mat and in chairs

Practice Ideas

Grounding Meditation

Grounding is the sensation of feeling connected to the earth, to being in our bodies, and to feeling safe. A grounding meditation may begin with noticing what you're experiencing externally through the senses, and then slowly shifting to noticing what's happening inside the body through interoception. This is a trauma-sensitive approach to meditation, and it would begin slowly with the external awareness first, exploring sight, hearing, touch, smell and taste. If that feels comfortable, then students can move their awareness inward to notice the breath, the heartbeat, and energy.

Imagery can be used in grounding meditations, but as I've mentioned previously, it's usually most helpful to stick to very general images. Specific images such as rushing water or wind in the trees might bring up disturbing memories for some people.

Breath Meditation

The most universal focus for meditation is the breath itself. The breath is always here, and most importantly, the breath is always in the present moment. By focusing on the breath, the mind is brought back into the present, which is the only time where we can actually feel happiness and peace.

When focusing on the breath, the mind can observe the physical sensations of breathing, such as cool air entering the nostrils and warmer air leaving; or focus on the energetic experience of the breath moving up and down the spine; or focus on the feeling of the whole body expanding on the inhale and contracting on the exhale.

Remember that while the breath is a constant, it may not be enjoyable for all students to focus on it. If they have a breathing disorder such as asthma, Long COVID, or chronic obstructive pulmonary disease, or if they have anxiety or trauma, focusing on the breath may actually trigger discomfort.

Earth & Sky Meditation

This is similar to a grounding meditation as you're focusing on the feeling of gravity, which is an ever-present force in our lives. First, explore the experience of gravity pulling the body toward the earth. (This practice can be most effective when done in shavasana, noticing all the points where the body is in contact with the floor, props, chair, or bed.) See if you can connect this supportive anchoring with the exhale.

Then, notice how the breath and prana (energy) in the body is lifting you away from the earth, toward the sky, in a dynamic rebound effect. See if you can connect this experience with the inhale. Continue to connect the exhale to grounding into the earth, and the inhale to lifting away toward the sky. You can visualize this energy flowing along the spine if that's helpful. If you like you can also repeat "earth" on the exhale, and "sky" on the inhale.

"Yes" Meditation

As an alternative to a traditional mantra or breath meditation, you can try allowing the mind to wander, while keeping part of the mind aware and conscious. To do this practice, see if you can notice every time a thought enters the mind, and then say the word, "yes." This practice will train your mind to observe itself without criticism. In fact, "yes" is a celebration of the mind's ability to think. Thoughts include words, images, and feelings. This technique can be an effective way to explore the power and capability of the mind without setting up an oppositional relationship with it. Spend a few minutes saying "yes" whenever you notice a thought. Then stop and notice how you're feeling.

Visual Meditation—*Trataka*

For students who are more visually inclined, there are ways to practice meditation with a visual focus. Traditionally, a candle flame, a flower, picture of a deity, or a mandala would be used, but you don't need any of those things to practice. In fact, staring at a point on the floor or the wall in front of you can be extremely effective.

Visual meditation can be used as a support for other meditation techniques, or by itself. If you're using it by itself, you can try focusing on the object for a brief period, and then close your eyes and picture the object in the mind. For example, when focusing on a light, you can also feel that light reflected within you. Visual meditations are often very effective for beginning meditators, or anyone for whom traditional meditation might be contraindicated.

Another form of visual meditation can be done by unfocusing your eyes and becoming aware of your entire field of vision at the same time, especially your peripheral vision. This is an effective technique when in nature or looking out a window.

"Who am I?" Meditation

Jnana Yoga, the path of wisdom, focuses on using the mind's own intelligence to transcend itself. That means that you use the mind's own ability to question in a reflective way. This isn't the path for everyone, but it can be a surprisingly effective technique for many students.

You can practice by repeating the question, "Who am I?" over and over in your mind. Occasionally, stop and listen for an answer. Alternatively, this is an effective guided meditation that you can lead for your students, where you ask them a series of questions very slowly, such as, "Am I the body? Am I the breath? Am I the thoughts? Where do the thoughts come from? Where do they go? Am I the mind? Who am I?"

Mantra Meditation

Practicing mantra repetition is a key element of yoga practice and is called *Japa Yoga*. Traditional Sanskrit mantras are sound vibrations that can be used to focus the mind. There are certain short mantras that are called *bija* mantras, or seed sounds.[112] They form the heart of longer mantras and are considered to be particularly powerful. In the end, all mantras are aspects of the cosmic hum, which is represented by the sound, "Om."

If a student has a devotional nature, they can explore the relationships between different Hindu deities and their related mantras. Or, they can focus on a universal mantra such as "Om Shanti," "Hari Om," or "Om Namah Shivaya." Of course, "Om" by itself is an incredibly powerful mantra.

Words from other languages can also be used, such as "peace" in English or "shalom" in Hebrew. Focusing on a particular word and repeating it can be a useful way to keep the mind focused. Also, encourage students to spend time exploring different mantras to see which feels best and resonates in their heart.

There are a number of techniques that support mantra repetition. My favorite one is to repeat the mantra out loud, and then get quieter and quieter, whispering the mantra, or even moving the lips without sound. As the mind gets more focused try moving into silence continuing to repeat it mentally.

Students can also coordinate the mantra with their breath in any way that feels comfortable. For example, they can repeat "Om" on the inhale, and repeat it again on the exhale. Or they can repeat a longer mantra just on the exhale. They can explore different ways to integrate their breath and chosen mantra. Mala beads are also incredibly helpful with mantra meditation.

They could also coordinate the mantra "So Ham" with their breath. This special mantra has a dual meaning. It represents the sound of the breath, and also means, "I am that," referring to the eternal unchanging spirit. On the inhale, repeat (or hear) "So" and on the exhale, repeat (or hear) "Ham."

Using a Mala

The use of prayer beads, or a mala, can be very helpful in making meditation accessible. A traditional mala is a string of 108 beads with a large knot, or *mehru*, at the end. This knot represents the divine. Some versions of traditional malas have a factor of 108 beads, such as 54 or 27, which can work for a bracelet mala.

There are a number of traditions regarding the use of a mala that are important to be aware of, whether or not your students are able to follow them. Generally, a mala is not considered jewelry or adornment, but a sacred object for spiritual practice. So it is traditionally kept private. For example, it would usually be worn under your shirt instead of on top of it. Also, you wouldn't let it touch the ground, and you would practice using the right hand. Traditionally, in South Asia, the right hand is considered cleaner than the left and is generally used for spiritual practices.

To use a mala:

- Raise your right hand in front of your heart with the palm facing you.
- Extend the index finger, and let the mala hang over the middle finger.
- Use the thumb to hold the mala against the middle finger and use the tip of the thumb to select a bead just above the mehru (the knot).
- As you repeat your mantra, such as "Om," you pull a bead toward you. Continue with your mantra repetition, pulling one bead toward you for each time you repeat the mantra.

If you do enough repetitions to end up at the mehru again, it's traditional to rotate the mala by flipping it around on your thumb and going back the other way. The mehru represents the divine, and it's not used like a regular bead. Similarly, the index finger represents the ego, and traditionally, you don't touch the mala with that finger.

To make the practice accessible, it's important to understand the underlying purpose of the mala and adapt the use of it in a way that is still respectful to the practice and also effective for you personally. For example, if you don't have use of your right hand, or you have arthritis in your hand, it is fine to find another hand position or to use the left hand.

Scenario

A student approaches you after class and says, "I like yoga but during the meditation my mind goes to some really dark places. Should I stop doing it?"

Response

It's great that this student feels comfortable enough with you to share their experience. I would suggest that they find a meditation technique that feels more uplifting, or simply not practice. There are some contraindications to meditation and they need to be taken seriously.[113] These problems usually occur in longer intensive meditations where people are sitting for hours on end. Generally, I don't think one minute of silence is very dangerous, but I always want my students to be comfortable and to have a positive experience.

This student might enjoy a visual meditation, keeping their eyes open and staring at a flower, candle, or a spot on the floor. They could also gaze out a window or at a photograph that is generally uplifting. Of course, they don't need to meditate, and they could choose to do something else instead. In their own practice, they might want to do more asana or pranayama.

Further Reflection

• What is your experience with meditation?

• Do you have a regular meditation practice, and if not, is that something you're interested in?

• How do you feel meditation connects to the other aspects of yoga that you teach?

• Can you find ways to incorporate meditation into your teaching?

EPILOGUE

My favorite role in yoga is that of an enthusiastic student. When I am immersed in the learning process I feel like I want to be a student forever. Each time that I teach it is a blessing to be able to share my enthusiasm with other students who are fellow seekers on the path. From the moment I stepped onto the yoga mat my deepest desire was just to practice. I never set out to be a yoga teacher as a career path. Instead, at some moment, it felt more like I answered the call of other students who needed support for their own journeys.

Teachers have a responsibility to be present and committed to all levels of students. Unfortunately, it's too easy for students to buy into a false equivalence between physical performance and spiritual development. In order for students and teachers to be fully engaged and inclusive, this misconception needs to be unpacked and unlearned. We need to understand that yoga is not the asanas, but that the asanas are tools, albeit powerful ones, to be used in service of yoga.

—Kino MacGregor

I JUST WANT TO SAY thank you for reading this book, and thank you for any effort you make to create more welcoming and accessible yoga spaces. Every single student matters, and every teacher as well. With one student at a time and one teacher at a time, we can really make a difference in the yoga community and potentially in the world.

As a teacher, your personal efforts to pull together what might feel like a lot of different threads and ideas will allow you to weave together a stronger community of practice, touching more and more lives along the journey. Each of us is like a single thread woven into a large ornate fabric. Individually, we may feel insignificant, but together we can create something truly beautiful.

Through our combined efforts, we can have an exponential impact on the way yoga is taught and practiced today. We can begin to center those of us who have so often been left on the outside of a practice that is based on universality. My prayer is that accessible yoga simply becomes yoga—and that it is the new norm.

The yoga teachings are very clear: We all share the same spirit, and the practice is designed to give us the direct experience of that universal oneness. We may not be able to experience it in every aspect of our lives, but at least in the context of our yoga classes, let's come together as one even as we celebrate our individuality and differences. That's the paradox of it all: The more we can celebrate our differences, the more we experience our interconnectedness.

I know that teaching yoga can be a challenging path in many ways. It can be hard to feel like you're knowledgeable enough, experienced enough, and truly prepared to take the seat of teacher. I hope this book helps to give you some more confidence to venture out into the world and share the practice you love, and to do so in a way that respects this beautiful tradition and is of service to the world.

To serve means to act from a place of love and care without focusing on your personal reward. It is yoga in action and one of the most challenging practices of all. Teaching yoga offers many opportunities for service. You get to care for others in a way that supports them on their journey, and most of all, in a way that supports your continued growth.

When you put yourself out into the world as a yoga teacher, you are forced to honestly look at yourself. Challenges will come that provide new learning opportunities. Ultimately that is a huge gift because teaching offers you a way to deepen your practice. As Kino MacGregor explained above, at the heart of every teacher is a dedicated student. You can allow your teaching to be a continuous education in itself if you're willing to learn from your students and your experiences.

Many blessings for your successful practice and teaching. As it says in this traditional peace chant from the *Taittiriya Upanishad,* may you be protected, nourished, and may you find peace.

Om saha navavatu saha nau bhunaktu
Saha viryam karavavahai
Tejasvi navadhitamastu
Ma vidvishavahai
Om shanti, shanti, shanti

Om, may we all be protected
May we all be nourished
May we work together with great energy
May our intellect be sharpened (may our study be effective)
Let there be no animosity amongst us
Om, peace, peace, peace[114]

GLOSSARY

ableism—Discrimination based on disability. The false belief that disabled people need to be fixed and healed.

Accessible Yoga—The name of an approach to yoga created by Jivana Heyman.

adaptive yoga—A general term for adjusting yoga practice to the student.

adho mukha svanasana—Downward facing dog pose.

ahimsa—The first of the five aspects of *yama*, the first limb of *ashtanga yoga*. *Ahimsa* means non-harm or nonviolence.

anandamaya kosha—The bliss body.

annamaya kosha—The physical body, or literally the body of food.

aparigraha—Non-attachment or non-greed.

ardha matsyendrasana—Half spinal twist, literally "half lord of the fishes pose."

Arjuna—The protagonist of the Bhagavad Gita. He is a great warrior and the leader of the Pandava brothers.

arthritis—The term refers to joint pain or joint disease, and there are more than 100 types of arthritis and related conditions including osteoarthritis, which is based on degradation of the joint, and rheumatoid arthritis which is an autoimmune disease that affects the joints.

asana—Yoga posture or pose.

ashtanga yoga—The eight limbs of yoga as described in Patanjali's Yoga Sutras in sutra 2.29. These include yama, niyama, asana, pranayama, pratyahara, dharana, dhyana, and samadhi.

Ashtanga Yoga—This is the name of a specific school of yoga created by Patabhi Jois.

asmita—A Sanskrit word for ego, specifically the feeling of having a separate identity, or I-am-ness.

asteya—The third aspect of yama. Asteya means not stealing, or generosity.

Atman—Refers to the individual spirit within each of us.

Bhagavad Gita—Indian scripture that is a part of the larger epic, the Mahabharata. The Gita tells the story of Arjuna being counseled by Krishna on how to be a yoga practitioner. Written approximately 2,000 years ago.

bhakti yoga—The devotional practices of yoga, such as mantra, *kirtan* (chanting), prayer, having a specific deity or image of the divine.

bhastrika—Bellow's breath. Similar to kapalabhati where there is equal force on the inhale and exhale.

bhujangasana—Cobra pose.

bitilasana—Cow pose.

brahmacharya—The fourth aspect of yama. The term brahmacharya traditionally meant celibacy, but is often translated in more contemporary times as conscious use of energy or resources.

brahmana—A term from ayurveda that means expansion, and is connected to the inhalation.

Brahmin—The priest caste in India.

Brihadaranyaka Upanishad—One of the principal Upanishads created around 700 BCE.

caste—The caste system is a type of hereditary social stratification based on rigid social groups.

casteism—Discrimination based on the caste system.

chitta—Term used by Patanjali to refer to the larger container of the mind.

debraminize—To remove caste and casteism.

dharana—The sixth limb of ashtanga yoga. Dharana means concentration, and is often described as the main practice of yoga meditation: focusing the mind on one thing.

dhyana—The seventh limb of ashtanga yoga. Dhyana means meditation, and describes the mental state that occurs in meditation, when the mind is connected to one focus.

garudasana—Eagle pose.

guru tattva—The essence of the guru, or the divine principle.

Hanh, Thich Nhat—A Vietnamese Buddhist monk who is known for his activism and social justice work. He founded the Plum Village Monastery in France.

hatha yoga—Refers to the physical practice of yoga.

Hatha Yoga Pradipika—A key historical text from the 15th century by Svatmarama detailing the physical practices of yoga.

HIV/AIDS—HIV (human immunodeficiency virus) is the virus that causes AIDS (acquired immunodeficiency syndrome).

Integral Yoga—The school of yoga founded in the United States by Swami Satchidananda, headquartered in Yogaville, Virginia.

interoception—A lesser-known sense that helps you understand and feel what's going on inside your body.

janushirshasana—Head to knee pose.

japa yoga—Mantra repetition.

jnana yoga—The wisdom practices of yoga, usually focused on self-inquiry.

Kabir—A fifteenth-century Indian mystic poet.

kapalabhati—Skull shining breath.

karma—Action and the result of action.

karma yoga—The path of selfless action often expressed through service, also called *seva*.

klesha—Mental affliction or obstacle.

kosha—Sheath, layer, or body.

krama—A step-by-step approach to asana.

Krishna—The teacher of Arjuna in the Bhagavad Gita, who is an incarnation of God.

langhana—From ayurveda. Means reduction, and refers to a calming practice that comes from lengthening the exhalation.

mala beads—Traditional prayer beads used to count mantras in the practice of japa yoga.

manomaya kosha—The mental body.

marjaryasana—Cat pose.

matsyasana—Fish pose.

mehru—The large bead with a tassel at the end of a mala. Also called the guru bead.

mudra—A gesture or position usually done with the hands that connects with subtle energy.

multiple sclerosis—A potentially disabling disease of the brain and spinal cord (central nervous system). In MS, the immune system attacks the protective sheath (myelin) that covers nerve fibers and causes communication problems between your brain and the rest of your body.

Nachiketa—The protagonist in the Katha Upanishad, who has a dialogue with Yama, the Lord of Death.

nadi shuddhi—Also known as nadi shodhana, nadi shodhanam, aniloma viloma, or sukha purvaka, refers to alternate nostril breathing.

nirodha—Restraint, calm, or stillness.

niyama—The second limb of ashtanga yoga, which means observances.

osteoporosis—A bone disease that develops when bone mineral density and bone mass decreases, or when the quality or structure of bone changes. This can lead to a decrease in bone strength that can increase the risk of broken bones.

panchamaya kosha—Five layers, bodies, or sheaths. Refers to the concept of human beings being made up of five layers: annamaya kosha, the physical body; pranamaya kosha, the breath/energy body; manomaya kosha, the mental body; vijnanamaya kosha, the wisdom body; and anandamaya kosha, the bliss body.

parsva sukhasana—Seated side bend.

Patanjali—The author of the Yoga Sutras, a demi-god who much of the teaching of yoga is attributed to.

prakriti—Creation.

pranamaya kosha—The energy or breath body.

pratyahara—The fifth limb of ashtanga yoga, which means withdrawal of the senses.

pranayama—The fourth limb of ashtanga yoga, which means breathing practices, or the expansion of energy.

proprioception—The sense that lets us perceive the location, movement, and action of parts of the body. It encompasses a complex of sensations, including perception of joint position and movement, muscle force, and effort.

Purusha—Spirit or true Self.

raja yoga—Historically meant the meditative goal of yoga, but often used as a synonym for the practice of Patanjali's yoga, or ashtanga yoga.

range of motion (ROM)—Means the extent or limit to which a part of the body can be moved around a joint or a fixed point; the totality of movement a joint is capable of doing.

samadhi—The eighth, and final, limb of ashtanga yoga, which means enlightenment, or super consciousness.

samskaras—Mental impressions, recollections, or psychological imprints.

Sanatana dharma—The eternal teachings that are at the heart of the yoga path. Later these teachings came to be referred to as Hinduism.

santosha—The second aspect of niyama, which means contentment.

Satchidananda, Swami—The founder of the school Integral Yoga.

satya—The second aspect of yama, which means truthfulness.

saucha—The first aspect of niyama, which means purity.

shavasana—The corpse pose, or relaxation pose.

seva—Service or karma yoga.

Shiva—Whose name means "the auspicious one," is part of the Hindu trinity of gods, including Brahma and Vishnu. He is called "the Destroyer."

stroke—Sometimes called a brain attack, occurs when something blocks blood supply to part of the brain or when a blood vessel in the brain bursts.

sukhasana—Easy pose, a cross-legged pose with the feet crossed at the ankles.

svadhyaya—The second aspect of kriya yoga, and the fourth niyama, which means self-study, study of the Vedas, recitation of mantra, or recitation of the Vedas.

tapas—The first aspect of kriya yoga, and the third niyama, which means purification, discipline, asceticism, or learning from suffering.

trataka—Gazing or visual meditation.

ujjayi—Whispering breath, ocean breath or, literally, victorious breath.

universal design—Creating an environment so that it can be accessed, understood, and used by all people, rather than expecting individuals to adapt to the environment.

upanishads—A group of ancient texts that form the end of the Vedas, and are offered as dialogues on spirituality.

utkata konasana—Goddess pose.

uttanasana—Standing forward bend.

utthita parsvakonasana—Extended side angle pose.

vairagya—Non-attachment, or literally, "without color."

Vedanta—One of the six schools of Hindu philosophy, focusing on the teachings of the Upanishads.

Vedas—A large body of ancient Indian scripture, including some of the oldest texts written in an Indo-European language. There are four Vedas: Rig Veda, Yajurveda, Samaveda, and Atharaveda, which are then each divided into four subsections including the Upanishads.

vijnanamaya kosha—The wisdom or intuitive body.

virabhadrasana 1—Warrior 1 pose.

virabhadrasana 2—Warrior 2 pose.

viveka kyathi—Discriminative discernment.

vritti—Thought and emotion, or the movement and disturbances of the mind.

vrksasana—Tree pose.

white supremacy—The belief (and systems that support it) that white people are superior than other races. The beliefs that support systemic racism and other forms of related oppression.

yama—The first limb of ashtanga yoga, which means abstention.

Yama—The Lord of Death, who is the teacher of Nachiketa in the Katha Upanishad.

Yoga Sutras of Patanjali (*Patanjalayogashastra*)—The text that is often considered the leading source of information for yoga philosophy, although there is some debate about how that came to be. The text includes 195 aphorisms, or short lessons, on how to practice yoga and attain levels of enlightenment. It was written approximately 400 CE.

CONTRIBUTORS

Amber Karnes (she/her) is a community builder, teacher, and writer based in Baltimore, Maryland. Her work is about creating accessible community spaces where folks can be themselves, stay curious, and take up more space in their own lives. Amber is the creator of Body Positive Yoga and the co-creator of the Accessible Yoga School. Her current project, amberhouse, is a developing collaboration with the youth of Baltimore bike life that helps teens realize their own personal power through bikes, art, and self-expression.

Anjali Rao (she/her) is a yoga practitioner-educator offering a multidisciplinary approach to sharing the teachings of yoga, integrating history, storytelling and art. She is a cancer survivor, and Indian American immigrant. She serves as the president of the Board of Directors of the Accessible Yoga Association and the host of *The Love of Yoga* podcast.

Avery Janeczek Kalapa (they, them) is a Certified Iyengar Yoga Teacher, community weaver at Sadhana Support Collective, and queer + trans wellness organizer; they are also an eRYT500, YACEP, BFA, with over two decades of yoga experience. Celebrated for their enthusiasm, devotion, and depth of somatic technique, Avery specializes in functional asana grounded in applied yoga philosophy. They support queers and other counter-culture yoga lovers to break the burn-out cycle and be nourished, and spiritually powerful without bypassing the wisdom of their body and lived experience. Avery's a parent, gardener, artist, creator; a white, queer, trans, nonbinary settler based in unceded Tiwa land, Albuquerque NM.

Indu Arora (she/her) is a yoga and Ayurveda teacher, mentor, and author, based in the U.S. Indu has been sharing about yoga philosophy, yoga therapy, and Ayurveda for the past two decades worldwide. She is inspired by and taught Kriya Yoga, Himalayan Yoga, Kashmir Shiavism, and Sivananda Yoga lineages. She has studied in a traditional Guru-Shishya parampara setting. Her core philosophy is "Yoga is a work-in and not a work-out." She is the author of *Mudra: The Sacred Secret* (2015), *Yoga: Ancient Heritage, Tomorrow's Vision* (2005, 2019), and *SOMA: 100 Heritage Recipes for Self-Care* (e-book, 2020; updated hard copy, 2022).

Jason Crandell (he/him) is a teacher by nature and author with more than 20 years of experience. Named "one of the teachers shaping the future of yoga," by *Yoga Journal*, Jason has been an in-demand teacher at conferences around the world for more than a decade. Considered a teacher's teacher, Jason has served as faculty in countless teacher trainings, faculties, leads trainings globally, and regularly presents teacher-training content at esteemed conferences.

Judith Hanson Lasater, PhD, PT, has taught yoga since 1971 in almost every state of the U.S. as well as on six continents. She is a founder of *Yoga Journal* magazine and the author of 11 books on yoga, the latest of which is *Teaching Yoga with Intention* (Shambhala, 2022).

Kino MacGregor (she/her) is a Miami native who is happiest on the beach with a fresh coconut. She is a poet at heart who always stops to smell the flowers. Kino is the founder of Omstars—the world's first yoga TV network. With over 1 million followers on Instagram and over 800,000 subscribers on YouTube and Facebook, Kino's message of spiritual strength reaches people all over the world. She's sought after worldwide as an expert yoga teacher and inspirational speaker. Kino is the author of four books, podcaster, and co-founder of Miami Life Center.

M Camellia (they/them) is a yoga practitioner and facilitator, writer, consent educator, and advocate called to create profoundly accessible spaces for self-inquiry. M is a co-founder of the Trans Yoga Project and, among other roles within the realm of yoga service, serves on the staff of the Accessible Yoga School. Their teaching and writing center Queer and Trans identity, consent and agency, body liberation, and disability justice in relation to yoga philosophy and practice. They serve as a mentor for other yoga teachers and practitioners who desire to deepen their understanding of accessibility, power dynamics, trauma, and yoga as social justice.

Melissa Shah (she/they) is an Indian-American yoga therapist who skillfully adapts yoga and Ayurveda to the individual. She grew up practicing yoga and believes that yoga doesn't need to be stripped of its culture and history in order for it to be palatable and beneficial to others. She is dedicated to the intersection of yoga and social justice and works to make feeling well accessible to all. With over 2000 hrs in training, they currently offer group and 1:1 yoga therapy and mentorships, retreats, and an online membership for those who want to practice anytime, anywhere.

Michelle Cassandra Johnson (she/her) is an author, activist, spiritual teacher and practitioner, racial equity consultant and trainer, and intuitive healer. Michelle teaches workshops and immersions and leads retreats and transformative experiences nationwide the focus on exploring embodied approaches to racial equity work, creating ritual in justice spaces, our divine connection with nature and Spirit, and how we as a culture can heal. Michelle is the author of *Skill in Action*, *Finding Refuge*, *We Heal Together,* published by Shambhala Publications, and *A Space For Us,* published by Beacon Press.

Nityda Gessel (she/her) is a somatic psychotherapist, trauma specialist, yoga teacher and educator, mom and heart-centered activist. Nityda is the founder of the Trauma-Conscious Yoga Institute, creator of The Trauma-Conscious Yoga Method℠, and author of *Embodied Self Awakening: Somatic Practices for Trauma Healing and Spiritual Evolution* (W. W. Norton & Company, 2023). Nityda has devoted her life to supporting the upliftment of others, working at the intersection of Eastern spirituality, holistic mental health, and embodied activism. Nityda founded the Trauma-Conscious Equity Foundation to narrow the health disparity gap by providing funding for BIPOC and LGBTQIA+ mental health professionals to receive yoga and somatic training.

Shanna Small (she/her) is a writer and yoga teacher who speaks to the intersectionality of yoga and social justice. She has practiced Ashtanga Yoga and studied the Yoga Sutras since 2001. Shanna finds joy in making yoga accessible for all. She is a contributor for Yoga International, OmStars, OmPractice and Embodied Philosophy. You can also find her online at Shanna Small Yoga. Shanna teaches trainings and workshops on diversity and inclusivity, the Yoga Sutras, and accessibility. She is a founding member of Yoga For Recovery Foundation, a nonprofit that helps those recovering from addiction, trauma, and systemic oppression.

Shawn Moore (he/him) Resides at the intersection of leadership and mindfulness. Shawn creates sacred spaces for stillness and self-inquiry to help changemakers align their strengths, intention, and impact. Through his integrative approach—which includes meditation, sound healing, yoga nidra, restorative yoga, and coaching—he holds transformative containers for self-renewal, personal discovery, and capacity-building that ease clients on their journey towards peace, clarity, and freedom.

Tracee Stanley (she/her) is the author of the bestselling book *Radiant Rest: Yoga Nidra for Deep Relaxation and Awakened Clarity* and the *The Luminous Self: Sacred Yogic Practices & Rituals to Remember Who You Are*. Tracee is the founder of Empowered Life Circle, a sacred community and portal of practices, rituals, and Tantric teachings inspired by more than 25 years of studentship in Sri Vidya Tantra and the teachings of the Himalayan Masters. Tracee is devoted to sharing the wisdom of yoga nidra, rest, meditation, self-inquiry, nature as a teacher, and ancestor reverence.

Tristan Katz (they/he) is a writer, educator, digital strategist, and equity-inclusion facilitator. They offer training and consulting on gender equity, trans inclusion, queer competency, and justice-focused marketing practices. Tristan's intention is to share this work with an anti-oppression and intersectional lens. He's worked with organizations and clients such as Kripalu Center for Yoga & Health, Accessible Yoga School, HubSpot, Stanford University's YogaX program, and Williston Northampton School, among many others. Tristan was named one of *Yoga Journal*'s 2021 Game Changers and is proud to serve on the Board of Directors of Accessible Yoga.

NOTES

1. Eknath Easwaran, *The Bhagavad Gita,* (Tomales, CA: Nilgiri Press, 2007), sloka 2.20.
2. Seth Powell, "The Ancient Yoga Strap," *The Luminescent*, June 2018, https://www.theluminescent.org/2018/06/the-ancient-yoga-strap-yogapatta.html.
3. Juan Mascaró, *The Upanishads,* (London: Penguin Books, 1965), Chandogya 8.1.
4. Swami Satchidananda, *The Living Gita: The Complete Bhagavad Gita,* (New York: Henry Holt & Co, 1990), sloka 2.7.
5. Swami Satchidananda, *The Yoga Sutras of Patanjali,* (Yogaville, VA: Integral Yoga Publications, 2003), sutra 1.3.
6. Swami Satchidananda, *The Yoga Sutras of Patanjali*, sutra 1.4.
7. Ashleigh Shackelford, "Fat Is Not a Bad Word," *Teen Vogue*, August 26, 2019, https://www.teenvogue.com/story/fat-is-not-a-bad-word.
8. Swami Satchidananda, *The Yoga Sutras of Patanjali*, sutra 2.6.
9. U.S. Department of Labor, Americans with Disabilities Act of 1990. Public Law 101-336. 108th Congress, 2nd session (July 26, 1990), https://www.dol.gov/general/topic/disability/ada.
10. Centers for Disease Control and Prevention, "Disability Impacts All of Us", Last Reviewed: May 15, 2023, https://www.cdc.gov/ncbddd/disabilityandhealth/infographic-disability-impacts-all.html.
11. "Yoga Mantras," Tummee, accessed on August 2, 2023, https://www.tummee.com/yoga-mantras.
12. Eliza Griswold, "Yoga Reconsiders the Role of the Guru in the Age of #MeToo," The New Yorker, July 23, 2019, https://www.newyorker.com/news/news-desk/yoga-reconsiders-the-role-of-the-guru-in-the-age-of-metoo.
13. Kristen Rogers, "Dear anti-racist allies: Here's how to respond to microaggressions," CNN, June 6, 2020, https://www.cnn.com/2020/06/05/health/racial-microaggressions-examples-responses-wellness/index.html.
14. Swami Satchidananda, *The Yoga Sutras of Patanjali*, sutra 2.31.

15. "Scope of Practice," Yoga Alliance, accessed on August 2, 2023, https://www.yogaalliance.org/Portals/0/policies/Scope_Of_Practice_yoga_Alliance.pdf.

16. "Scope of Practice for Yoga Therapy," International Association of Yoga Therapists,September1,2020,https://cdn.ymaws.com/www.iayt.org/resource/resmgr/docs_certification_all/2020_updates_scope_ethics/2020-09_sop_v2.pdf.

17. "Sanskrit Chants," Yogaville, accessed on August 28, 2023, https://www.yogaville.org/sanskrit-chants/.

18. P. S. Sundaram, *The Kural*, (India: Penguin Books, 1990), verse 350.

19. Joshua J. Mark, "Upanishads," World History Encyclopedia, June 10, 2020, https://www.worldhistory.org/Upanishads/.

20. Swami Krishnananda, *The Brihadaranyaka Upanishad*, The Divine Life Society, accessed on August 31, 2023, https://www.swami-krishnananda.org/brdup/brhad_V-01.html, verse 4.4.5.

21. Eknath Easwaran, *The Upanishads*, (Tomales, CA: Nilgiri Press, 2007), Katha Upanishad, verse 2.3.13.

22. Ibid., Isha Upanishad, verse 6-7.

23. Swami Satchidananda, *The Living Gita*, sloka 2.48.

24. Ibid., sloka 6.22-26, 2.50.

25. Ibid., sloka 2.41.

26. Ibid., sloka 12.19.

27. Easwaran, *The Bhagavad Gita,* sloka 3.25.

28. Ibid., sloka 6.19.

29. A. G. Mohan & Dr. Ganesh, *Hatha Yoga Pradipika: Translation with Notes from Krishnamacharya* (Svastha yoga, 2017), verse 1.10.

30. Ibid., verse 1.12.

31. Ibid., verse 1.64.

32. Ibid., verse 2. 2.

33. Ibid., verse 2.15.

34. Brian Dana Akers, *The Hatha Yoga Pradipika*, YogaVidya.com, 002. https://www.yogavidya.com/Yoga/hatha-yoga-pradipika.pdf, chapter 2.29.

35. Ibid., chapter 3.1-2.

36. Ibid., chapter 4.5-6.

37. Ibid., chapter 4.55-59.

38. Michele Marie Desmarais, *Changing Minds: Mind, Consciousness and Identity in Patanjali's Yoga Sutra*, (Delhi: Motilal Banarsidass, 2008), pages 16-17.

39. Swami Satchidananda, *The Yoga Sutras of Patanjali,* sloka 2.28.

40. Ibid., sloka 3.19-20.

41. Plum Village App Team, "A short guide to joining or starting a sangha," Plum Village, March 1, 2022, https://plumvillage.app/a-short-guide-to-joining-or-starting-a-sangha/.

42. Swami Satchidananda, The Living Gita, sloka 6.29.

43. Ibid., sloka 3.25-26.

44. M Camellia, "Creating Cultures of Consent in Yoga," *Accessible Yoga Blog,* April 28, 2022, https://www.accessibleyoga.org/blog/creating-cultures-of-consent-in-yoga.

45. Angela Carter, 1983, https://libquotes.com/angela-carter/quote/lba4s5m.

46. Thenmozhi Soundararajan, "The Trauma of Caste," Podcast Audio. *The Love of Yoga Podcast with Anjali Rao,* Season 4, episode 1. January 6, 2023, https://www.accessibleyoga.org/podcasts/the-love-of-yoga/episodes/2147844786.

47. Tara Haelle, "Identity-first vs. person-first language is an important distinction," *Association of Health Care Journalists,* July 31, 2019, https://healthjournalism.org/blog/2019/07/identity-first-vs-person-first-language-is-an-important-distinction/.

48. Pronouns.org: Resources on Personal Pronouns, accessed on August 4, 2023, https://pronouns.org/how.

49. RAINN (Rape, Abuse & Incest National Network), accessed on August 4, 2023, https://www.rainn.org/articles/sexual-harassment.

50. Ellis Carter, "The Pros and Cons of Fiscal Sponsorship," CharityLawyer, February 10, 2020, https://charitylawyerblog.com/2020/02/10/the-pros-and-cons-of-fiscal-sponsorship/.

51. Liam Stack, Katherine Rosman and Jan Ransom, "Yoga Chain Reaped Millions but Filed No Taxes for Years, Prosecutors Say," *New York Times,* August 24, 2022, https://www.nytimes.com/2022/08/24/nyregion/tax-fraud-yoga-to-the-people.html.

52. ARD (Anti-Racism Daily), accessed on August 4, 2023, https://the-ard.com/glossary/white-savior-complex/.

53. Linda Sparrowe, "Yoga & Cancer: A Healing Journey," *Accessible Yoga Blog,* October 7, 2022, https://www.accessibleyoga.org/blog/yoga-cancer-a-healing-journey.

54. "Yoga Teacher Liability Waiver," beYogi, accessed on August 4, 2023, https://beyogi.com/yoga-liability-waiver-ppc/.

55. Anne Asher, CPT, "What Is a Posterior Pelvic Tilt?," Verywell Health, March 5, 2023, https://www.verywellhealth.com/posterior-pelvic-tilt-297132.

56. Carmine Gallo, "The Maya Angelou Quote That Will Radically Improve Your Business," *Forbes,* May 31, 2014, https://www.forbes.com/sites/carminegallo/2014/05/31/the-maya-angelou-quote-that-will-radically-improve-your-business/.

57. Arnold YL Wong, Jaro Karppinen, and Dino Samartzis, "Low back pain in older adults: risk factors, management options and future directions," NIH National Library of Medicine, v.12; April 18, 2017, https://www.ncbi.nlm.nih.gov/pmc/articles/PMC5395891/.

58. Yoga for Arthritis, accessed on August 4, 2023, https://www.arthritis.yoga/

59. Jennifer D'Angelo Friedman, "What the Bikram Copyright Rejection Means for Yoga," *Yoga Journal*, October 16, 2015, https://www.yogajournal.com/lifestyle/yoga-trends/rejection-bikram-copyright-upheld-means-future-yoga/.

60. Kathy Zetterberg, "Is Static Stretching Effective for Injury Prevention?," NASM, accessed on August 29, 2023, https://blog.nasm.org/fitness/is-static-stretching-the-best-strategy-for-injury-prevention-and-performance-enhancement.

61. Natasha Freutel, "Stretching Exercises for Seniors to Improve Mobility," Health-line, October 16, 2019, https://www.healthline.com/health/senior-health/stretching-exercises.

62. "Adult Learning Theories," TEAL (Teaching Excellence in Literacy), accessed on August 4, 2023, https://lincs.ed.gov/sites/default/files/11_%20TEAL_Adult_Learning_Theory.pdf.

63. Wikipedia, accessed on August 4, 2023, https://en.wikipedia.org/wiki/Andragogy.

64. "Aging and the ADA," ADA National Network, accessed on August 28, 2023, https://adata.org/factsheet/aging-and-ada.

65. "Disability," WHO (World Health Organization), accessed on August 4, 2023, https://www.who.int/news-room/fact-sheets/detail/disability-and-health.

66. "1 in 4 US adults live with a disability," CDC (Centers for Disease Control and Prevention), August 16, 2018, https://www.cdc.gov/media/releases/2018/p0816-disability.html.

67. "Chair Yoga for Everyone: Learn to Practice & Teach," Accessible Yoga School, accessed on August 28, 2023, https://www.accessibleyogaschool.com/chair-yoga-for-everyone.

68. Matthew Sanford, "Trusting the Yoga," Podcast Audio, Accessible Yoga Podcast, Season 2, June 6, 2022, https://www.accessibleyoga.org/podcasts/the-love-of-yoga/episodes/2147743271.

69. Hailey Hudson, "Moving From Disability Rights to Disability Justice," WID (World Institute on Disability), accessed on August 4, 2023, https://wid.org/moving-from-disability-rights-to-disability-justice/.

70. Sins Invalid, accessed on August 4, 2023, https://www.sinsinvalid.org/.

71. "10 Principles of Disability Justice," Sins Invalid, September 17, 2015, https://www.sinsinvalid.org/blog/10-principles-of-disability-justice.

72. Amber Karnes, "Making Peace With Your Body," Podcast Audio, Accessible Yoga Podcast, Season 1: Episode 13, October 20, 2020, https://www.accessibleyoga.org/podcasts/the-love-of-yoga/episodes/2147576664.

73. Thomas A. Swain, MPH and Gerald McGwin, MS, PhD, "Yoga-Related Injuries in the United States From 2001 to 2014", NIH National Library of Medicine, v.4(11); 2016 Nov, https://www.ncbi.nlm.nih.gov/pmc/articles/PMC5117171/.

74. NIH (National Institute on Deafness and Other Communication Disorders), accessed on August 4, 2023, https://www.nidcd.nih.gov/health/age-related-hearing-loss.

75. Carol Krucoff, C-IAYT, E-RYT, "Some Commonly-Taught Yoga Poses May Present Risks for Older Adults," Duke Health and Well-Being, August 28, 2019, https://dhwblog.dukehealth.org/some-commonly-taught-yoga-poses-may-present-risks-for-older-adults/.

76. Kinsey Mahaffey, "The Rate of Perceived Exertion (RPE) Scale Explained," NASM, accessed on August 29, 2023, https://blog.nasm.org/rate-of-perceived-exertion.

77. Joseph Campbell, "The First Storytellers," Video Recording, The Power of Myth with Bill Moyers, Ep. 3, June 23, 1988, https://billmoyers.com/content/ep-3-joseph-campbell-and-the-power-of-myth-the-first-storytellers-audio/.

78. Holger Cramer, Daniela Quinker, Dania Schumann, Jon Wardle, Gustav Dobos, and Romy Lauche, "Adverse effects of yoga: a national cross-sectional survey," NIH National Library of Medicine, v.19; 2019 Jul, https://www.ncbi.nlm.nih.gov/pmc/articles/PMC6664709/.

79. Mayo Clinic, accessed on August 5, 2023, https://www.mayoclinic.org/diseases-conditions/foot-drop/symptoms-causes/syc-20372628.

80. Dr. Jennifer Cumming, "Sport Imagery Training," Association for Applied Sport Psychology, accessed on August 4, 2023, https://appliedsportpsych.org/resources/resources-for-athletes/sport-imagery-training/.

81. Dictionary.com, accessed on August 4, 2023, https://www.dictionary.com/browse/modification.

82. Amy Wheeler, Ph.D., "Yoga Practice: The Wisdom of Krama," YogaUOnline, June 17, 2014, https://yogauonline.com/yoga-practice-teaching-tips/yoga-practice-tips/yoga-practice-the-wisdom-of-krama/.

83. Martin Noon, "Adaptive Teaching: A Practical Step-by-Step Guide," Third Space Blog, June 27, 2023, https://thirdspacelearning.com/blog/adaptive-teaching/.

84. Dr. Gail Parker, Empowered by Yoga, accessed on August 4, 2023, https://www.drgailparker.com/.

85. Kathi Valeii, "How Does Intergenerational Trauma Work?," Verywell Health, September 4, 2021, https://www.verywellhealth.com/intergenerational-trauma-5191638.

86. Michelle Cassandra Johnson, We Heal Together, (Boulder, CO: Shambhala, 2023), page 83.

87. Easwaran, The Upanishads, Katha Upanishad 1.1.4.

88. Equality Labs, accessed on August 6, 2023, https://www.equalitylabs.org.

89. Easwaran, The Upanishads, Katha Upanishad 1.2.18, 1.2.22.

90. Kff.org, accessed on August 4, 2023, https://www.kff.org/coronavirus-covid-19/press-release/latest-federal-data-show-that-young-people-are-more-likely-than-older-adults-to-be-experiencing-symptoms-of-anxiety-or-depression/.

91. Indu Arora, "Restorative Yoga Series: Making Rest Practices Accessible," Online Course through The Accessible Yoga School, April 12, 2023, https://www.accessibleyogaschool.com/restorative-series.

92. Swami Satchidananda, *The Yoga Sutras of Patanjali*, sutra 2.52.

93. Ibid., sutra 2.5.

94. Robert Bly, *The Soul is Here for Its Own Joy,* (Hopewell, NJ: Ecco Press, 1995), page 88.

95. Nityda Gessel, *Embodied Self Awakening: Somatic Practices for Trauma Healing and Spiritual Evolution*, (New York: W. W. Norton & Co. 2023, pages 3-4.

96. "How Box Breathing Can Help You Destress," Cleveland Clinic, accessed on August 4, 2023, https://health.clevelandclinic.org/box-breathing-benefits/.

97. Kristen Rogers, "The 4-7-8 method that could help you sleep," CNN, March 14, 2023, https://www.cnn.com/2022/09/16/health/4-7-8-breathing-technique-relaxing-wellness/index.html.

98. Ieva Aleknaitė-Dambrauskienė, PhD, "How the Diaphragm Impacts Your Entire Body," Healthnews, April 3, 2023, https://healthnews.com/health-conditions/musculoskeletal-disorders/diaphragm-function-and-its-connection-with-other-organs/.

99. "Diaphragmatic Breathing," Cleveland Clinic, accessed on August 4, 2023, https://my.clevelandclinic.org/health/articles/9445-diaphragmatic-breathing.

100. Ellen O'Brien, "You May Be Able to Lower Your Risk of Alzheimer's Through Breathing Exercises, According to Researchers," *Yoga Journal*, May 23, 2023, https://www.yogajournal.com/lifestyle/alzheimers-slow-breathing-study/.

101. Rolf Sovik and Dick Ravizza, PhD, "Self-Study: Nostril Dominance," Yoga International, accessed on August 30, 2023, https://yogainternational.com/article/view/self-study-nostril-dominance/.

102. Kirsten Nunez, "7 Science-Backed Benefits of Pranayama," healthline, May 15, 2020, https://www.healthline.com/health/pranayama-benefits.

103. Morgana M. Novaes, Fernanda Palhano-Fontes, Heloisa Onias, Katia C. Andrade, Bruno Lobão-Soares, Tiago Arruda-Sanchez, Elisa H. Kozasa, Danilo F. Santaella, Draulio Barros de Araujo, "Effects of Yoga Respiratory Practice (Bhastrika pranayama) on Anxiety, Affect, and Brain Functional Connectivity and Activity: A Randomized Controlled Trial," *Frontiers*, May 21, 2020, https://www.frontiersin.org/articles/10.3389/fpsyt.2020.00467/full.

104. Ranil Jayawardena, Priyanga Ranasinghe, Himansa Ranawaka, Nishadi Gamage, Dilshani Dissanayake, and Anoop Misra, "Exploring the Therapeutic Benefits of Pranayama (Yogic Breathing): A Systematic Review," NIH National

Library of Medicine, v.13(2); May-Aug 2020, https://www.ncbi.nlm.nih.gov/pmc/articles/PMC7336946/.

105. Easwaran, *The Upanishads*, Shvetashvatara Upanishad 3:13, 4:4-5.

106. Swami Satchidananda, *The Yoga Sutras of Patanjali*, sutra 1.32.

107. Ibid., sutra 1.39.

108. Ibid., sutra 3.1.

109. "5 Surprising Benefits of Meditation," *Yoga Alliance Blog*, May 19, 2023, https://blog.yogaalliance.org/5-surprising-benefits-of-meditation/.

110. Easwaran, *The Upanishads,* Kena Upanishad 1.1-1.2, page 213.

111. "Meditation and Mindfulness: What You Need To Know," NIH National Center for Complementary and Integrative Health, June 2022, https://www.nccih.nih.gov/health/meditation-and-mindfulness-what-you-need-to-know.

112. Timothy Burgin, "Bija Mantras: Definition, Types and Benefits," Yoga Basics, October 13, 2022, https://www.yogabasics.com/connect/yoga-blog/bija-mantras/.

113. Sarah Simon, "Too Much Mindfulness Can Worsen Your Mental Health," Verywell Health, June 2, 2021, https://www.verywellhealth.com/mindfulness-can-be-harmful-researchers-say-5186740.

114. Jhula Yoga, accessed on August 30, 2023, https://jhulayogayork.wordpress.com/teacher/mantra-om-sahana-vavatu/.

INDEX

ABOUT THE AUTHOR

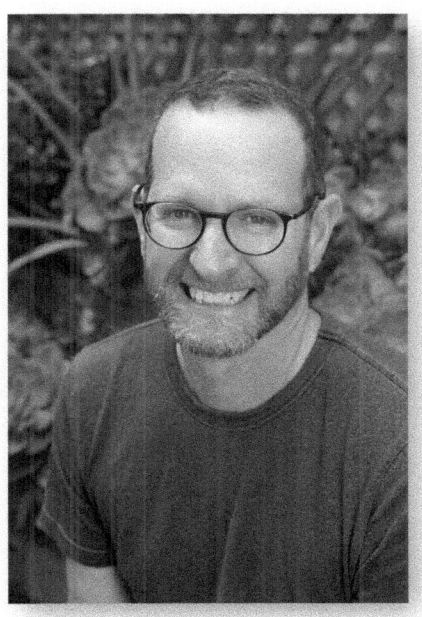

Jivana Heyman, C-IAYT, E-RYT 500, is the founder and director of the Accessible Yoga Association, an international nonprofit organization dedicated to increasing access to the yoga teachings. He's the author of *Accessible Yoga: Poses and Practices for Every Body*, and *Yoga Revolution: Building a Practice of Courage & Compassion*.

Jivana has specialized in sharing yoga with communities that have been excluded in contemporary yoga spaces. Out of this work, the nonprofit Accessible Yoga Association was created to support education, training, and advocacy with the mission of shifting the public perception of yoga. Jivana is also the creator of the Accessible Yoga Training and co-founder of the online Accessible Yoga School with Amber Karnes, which is a platform for continued education for yoga teachers in the field of equity and accessibility.

Jivana coined the phrase, "accessible yoga," over fifteen years ago, and it has become the standard appellation for a large cross section of the immense yoga world. He brought the Accessible Yoga community together for the first time in 2015 for the Accessible Yoga Conference.

He lives in Santa Barbara, California, with his husband, Matt. They have two grown children, Charlie and Violet. He also enjoys biking and gardening, and spending time with other yoga teachers.